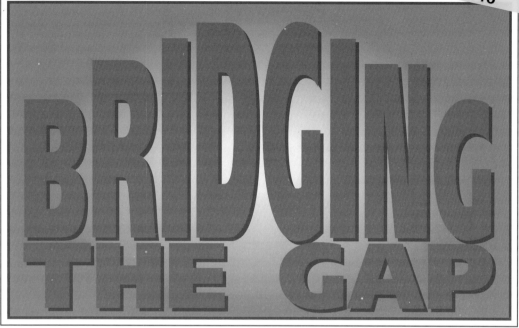

BRUCE BRADSHAW

Foreword by Paul G. Hiebert

INNOVATIONS
IN MISSION

Bryant L. Myers, Series Editor

BRIDGING THE GAP
Evangelism, Development and *Shalom*

Bruce Bradshaw

Unless otherwise noted, Scripture quotations are taken from the HOLY BIBLE, NEW INTERNATIONAL VERSION®. NIV®. Copyright © 1973, 1978, 1984 by International Bible Society. Used by permission of Zondervan Publishing House. All rights reserved.

ISBN 0-912552-84-0

Published by MARC, a division of World Vision International, 121 East Huntington Drive, Monrovia, California 91016-3400, U.S.A.

Printed in the United States of America. Editor and interior page layout: Edna Valdez. Cover design: Robbin Burrows.

Bridging the Gap is the fifth in MARC's Innovations In Mission series.

Other books in this series are:

The Nonresidential Missionary
Empowering the Poor
Facing the Powers
The Spirit Said "Grow"

CONTENTS

THE 1990s are a time of rapid change in almost every area of life. The political and economic maps are being redrawn. Technology is advancing at a dizzying pace. The center of gravity of Christ's body in the world has shifted to the southern hemisphere. The church is exploding in China and on the Pacific Rim. Theology of mission is being written at the grassroots among the poor. The cost of misusing and abusing God's creation is staring us in the face.

In the midst of this climate of rapid change, extreme complexity and almost obsessive pluralism, the church of Jesus Christ is to be in mission. The good news of Jesus Christ and the claims of his kingdom are needed everywhere.

Post-Christian Europe needs to rediscover the gospel that was once central to its culture and sense of being. The nomadic pastoralists—living across the Sahel in Africa, throughout the Middle East, in the eastern provinces of the former USSR and in western and southern China—need to hear a gospel "that will fit on the back of a camel." The poor in Latin America need a gospel that restores their relationship with God and reverses the erosion of their quality of life. North Americans need to hear a good news that restores vibrancy of worship and commitment to social change to their culturally captive brand of Christianity. The rich and powerful everywhere need to hear how difficult it is for them to get in the kingdom of heaven.

MARC is in the business of inspiring vision and motivating mission among those who are taking the whole gospel to the whole world. One of the ways we seek to fulfill our mission is to identify and share the stories of innovations in mission which, in our fallible view, make sense in this kind of changing, chaotic world. We seek to broadcast what we have discovered as good news in mission in hopes that others might find this information useful in enhancing their own mission. This series, *Innovations in Mission,* is the tool we have chosen for sharing this information with the global Christian mission community. We hope it will be valuable to mission strategists and executives, mission professors and students, and all those for whom Christian mission is part of living life with Christ.

Bridging the Gap is the fifth book in this series. Its subject is one of the most debilitating ideas of the last two centuries: the idea that there is an unbridgeable gap between the world of spiritual and religious things and the real world of science, development and technology. This dichotomy has led to the separation of evangelism and social action, public and private truth, values and facts, faith and reason. Accepting this view of reality, the church has accepted its banishment to the realm of the personal, private and interior, leaving the public and exterior world to the dehumanizing impact of modernity. This accommodation has shaped and disempowered Christian mission and separated brothers and sisters of faith.

Recognizing the problem is only the beginning. The critical and much harder question is how do we recover. Simply reuniting the two spheres is not enough. We have to do the hard work of recovering the seamless, inseparable, living understanding of the Bible in which the two were never meant to be separated in the first place.

Bruce Bradshaw, MARC's director of holistic development research, does this in *Bridging the Gap*. Approaching the problem from a critique of the Enlightenment two-tiered world view, he argues for a Biblical view and then demonstrates how it changes our understanding of management, education, environmentalism, economics, healing and coping with principalities and powers.

BRYANT L. MYERS
SERIES EDITOR

Foreword

NOTHING HAS HINDERED the modern mission movement more than modern dualism that separates body from spirit, science from religion, and natural from supernatural.

This dualism has led some to equate the Christian mission with an evangelism that seeks to save lost souls from eternal damnation, and leaves ministries to earthly human needs to secular agencies.

There is truth in this view. The gospel is indeed about eternal life in Jesus Christ, and heaven. But this view calls people to follow a distant, theological Christ who no longer walks the roads of life, one who saves us only after death. Many heard this gospel, and turned back to their old religions, because these offered them concrete answers to the crises of everyday life.

This view also led missionaries to ignore the sociocultural and historical contexts of the people they served. Consequently, the people did not hear the gospel in ways they could understand and believe. For them it was a foreign gospel of a god speaking to strangers in a distant land, not of a God who has come to save *them* in their setting.

Other missionaries focused on human needs, and proclaimed a gospel that promises food, healing, justice and a better life here on earth.

There is truth in this view as well. Christ came not only to die for our sins, but to inaugurate the kingdom of God on earth. He walked the roads with the common people, healing them, feeding them, and preaching justice. Above all he called them to follow him and become part of his church, the outpost of his kingdom on earth. But this, too, is a half gospel, for Christ did come to save us from damnation. We fail in our mission if we improve people's lives, but do not lead them to eternal life.

Attempts at presenting a holistic gospel

Seeing the truncated nature of these gospels, many missionaries sought to combine the two, preaching a message of spiritual salvation, and practicing a ministry of human well-being.

There is much to be said for this attempt at presenting a holistic gospel. Around the world churches were planted, and schools, hospitals

and agricultural programs established. The educational and medical programs in many countries have their roots in the great missionary movement of the nineteenth and early twentieth centuries.

This approach, however, had unforeseen consequences that weakened the life of the young churches. First, the pressing nature of human
needs in times of famine, plagues and oppression often led to a neglect of
the preaching of the message of eternal salvation. Most time and
resources were increasingly spent on maintaining Western-style schools,
hospitals and development programs.

A second consequence was the spread of modern dualism along
with the gospel. The people saw the church as fruit of the gospel, and
schools and hospitals as the products of science. But this only reflected
what was true in the minds of many Western missionaries. These missionaries preached the Bible in the churches. They taught the texts of science in schools and hospitals. These were not integrated in mission
because they were not integrated in the minds of the missionaries.

Many people believed the sciences, but rejected Christ, because
the sciences had direct relevance to their lives. Ironically, Christian missions became one of the great secularizing forces of the past century
around the world.

A more subtle form of this dualism was the argument that Christian agencies should carry out social ministries for their own sake, and not
with the intent to evangelize people, lest we produce "rice Christians."
One consequence of this dualism was the wedding of Christianity to
Western culture and the enlightenment notion of "progress."

The superiority of science over traditional beliefs seemed self-evi-
dent to Western Christians. They saw their mission to non-Western people
as bringing them Christianity, Civilization and Commerce. Missionaries
expected new converts to wear Western clothing, embrace Western medicine, and study in Western-style schools. The result was a colonial pater-
nalism that disempowered the people, and kept them from developing a
vital, indigenous form of Christianity in their own sociocultural contexts.

In recent years some missiologists have tried to get away from
modern dualism and its distortions of the gospel. The answer, they say, is
to reject the modern world view, and to adopt a Christian animism that
unites spiritual and natural realities. They escape the evils of Western
dualism, however, only to be captured by another pagan world view.

One form of animism is pantheism—all phenomenological realities are manifestations of one cosmic spirit. There is no god other than
nature itself. A second form is a distant high god, who, in anger at
human folly, has left humans to fend for themselves in a world of invisible spirits and forces. Both forms are totally antithetical to a Christian

world view because they, like modern science, are human-centered. In secular science, people seek to control their lives by means of empirical knowledge. In animism, they seek to control the gods, spirits and powers for their own purposes by means of sacred rites, magic, witchcraft, divination and sacrifices appeasement. Neither begins with God.

A biblical approach to holistic mission

While an animistic approach to Christianity seeks to restore to us a sense of God's work in our everyday lives, it perverts the very nature of the gospel and reduces it to a gospel of health and wealth. It makes us gods and lovers of ourselves (2 Tim. 3:1-5). A biblical approach to holistic mission is neither a modern dualism, nor a Christian animism. It is a third alternative that we need to rediscover.

In this pioneering work, Bruce Bradshaw charts the basic elements of a biblical view of holistic ministry. Building on the theological foundations of creation, redemption and *shalom*, he shows us how these encompass all areas of human life. In doing so, he avoids the common error of seeking theological principles to justify theories built on other foundations.

But this is no abstract theology of whole mission divorced from the realities of field ministries, a divorce that readmits modern dualism through the back door. Bradshaw's writing emerges out of difficult and profound reflections gleaned from his years of ministry. Using concrete cases, he examines the world views of the people and of the cross-cultural workers, and shows the flaws of both in the light of biblical truth. He then shows how a biblical approach can provide another answer to the needs of fallen humanity. Bradshaw does not avoid the complexities of human life, nor does he offer simplistic answers.

Some will disagree with the solutions Bradshaw offers. The value of his work, however, is not in the specific answers he gives, but in the fact that he has set the missiological foundations on which the debate must build. By calling us to re-examine the world view we bring to the theology and practice of mission, he helps us to see our deep cultural biases, and to read the Scriptures in the light of their own categories and assumptions. Out of this can emerge a new understanding of the full nature of God's great salvation.

Nor does Bradshaw reject what the modern sciences offer us in understanding humans and their sociocultural contexts. Rather, he critiques and reinterprets scientific insights in the light of biblical truth. In so doing he avoids another common dualism in our day, namely attempting to restore a sense of God's presence in human lives by rejecting what the sciences can teach us. Modern science is the child of Christianity and, restored again to its place in a truly biblical world view, it can help us greatly in holistic ministries.

The second value of Bradshaw's work is to help those of us in the Western church to see ourselves and our churches more clearly. Not only have modern dualism and animism harmed the modern mission movement, they have weakened the church in the West. A rediscovery of a biblical view of creation, sin, salvation and *shalom* would revitalize us and help us to live as the early Christians did, gathering in communities of *shalom*, proclaiming the good news of God's whole salvation, and transforming the world around them.

PAUL G. HIEBERT

Acknowledgments

I WANT TO THANK the many people who contributed to this book. I am indebted to many friends and colleagues at World Vision International who read the initial drafts. They provided valuable guidance, critiques and editorial expertise.

Friends and colleagues in World Vision field offices also provided information, stories and insights. I was humbled by the amount of guidance John Steward of World Vision Australia gave me. Comments from David Burns helped me clarify some critical issues. I also appreciated affirmation from two people I highly esteem, Paul Clasper and Lance Schaina. Paul Hiebert and Jayakumar Christian graciously offered their thoughts on the introductory chapters.

I also must mention Mary, Ellen, Amy and Phillip. Mary lent her husband, and the children lent their father to this book.

Introduction

In Lystra there sat a man crippled in his feet,
who was lame from birth and had never walked.
He listened to Paul as he was speaking.
Paul looked directly at him,
saw that he had faith to be healed and called out,
"Stand up on your feet!"
At that, the man jumped up and began to walk.

When the crowd saw what Paul had done, they shouted . . .
"The gods have come down to us in human form!". . .
The priest of Zeus . . . brought bulls . . .
to offer sacrifices to them.

But when the apostles Barnabas and Paul heard of this,
they . . . rushed into the crowd, shouting:
". . . We too are only men, human like you.
We are bringing you good news,
telling you to turn from
these worthless things to the living God,
who made heaven and earth and sea
and everything in them . . .
He has shown kindness by giving you
rain from heaven and crops in their seasons;
he provides you with plenty of food
and fills your hearts with joy."
Even with these words,
they had difficulty keeping the crowd
from sacrificing to them.
Acts 14:8-18

WHEN THE PEOPLE in Lystra saw Paul heal the lame man, they assumed
that Paul and Barnabas were incarnations of Hermes and Zeus, their local

gods. The Lystrans attributed the healing to these gods because of the basic assumptions they used to interpret reality. They responded to the presence of the gods by making sacrifices to them.

Paul saw the Lystrans preparing the sacrifices, and told them the good news of the living God. Because he interpreted reality differently, Paul believed the healing was the work of a different God. Paul portrayed this God as the Creator, Sustainer and Provider who made heaven, earth, the seas and everything in them. Paul affirmed that God gives rain from heaven and crops in their seasons.

Despite the persuasiveness of Paul's discourse, many Lystrans refused to change the basic assumptions about the healing they witnessed. They continued to believe that Paul and Barnabas were incarnations of Zeus and Hermes.

Our basic assumptions and Christian mission

Our basic assumptions about life comprise our world views. They have a profound impact on Christian mission. Consider the assumptions many Christians from Western cultures make about development work.

The assumptions of our Western world view lead us to separate the physical and spiritual dimensions of reality. In making this separation, we assume that redemption affects the spiritual instead of the physical realm. This view of redemption leads us to assume that development work does not make a direct spiritual contribution to Christian mission.

This assumption creates a need for us to justify why we feed the hungry, treat the sick, and educate the illiterate. Some of us justify development work because it creates opportunities for evangelism. Others say development complements evangelism like the two wings of a bird complement each other. Yet people who hold this view often do not extend it to seeing redemption in the physical realm.

Both positions are valid to some extent, but they miss two important points about Christian mission.

The first point is that Christian mission is an effort to express God's redemptive work in all creation. Colossians 1:15-20 impresses us with God's effort to reconcile the seen and unseen elements of creation to himself through Christ, thus bringing peace. We cannot bring the Good News of Jesus Christ to the ends of the earth without recognizing that redemption affects the fullness of creation.

The second point of Christian mission that we are prone to miss is the need to address the basic assumptions people make about life when we communicate the Good News.

To people in many parts of the world, the dichotomy between the physical and spiritual realms of creation that Western Christians make has little sense. These people have a primal world view. They do not assume we can split reality into two realms that do not normally interact. Instead, they see creation woven together as a seamless garment. They believe the spiritual realm governs the behavior of the physical realm. They do not believe the physical realm is self-sufficient. Rather, they believe that changes in the spiritual realm cause changes in the physical realm.

People with a primal world view ask different questions about the spirituality of development. They want to know the spiritual realm governs the changes we are attempting to make in the physical realm. Do we seek permission from the spiritual realm to make these changes? Have we performed the correct ceremonies or sacrifices to get the blessing of the spiritual realm? Where is God in the knowledge, expertise and technology we bring to their cultures? Is the power of Jesus stronger than the powers of the witch doctors or shamans?

The biblical world view bridges the gap

This book is an attempt to illustrate how the biblical world view offers an interpretation of reality that bridges the gap between the Western and primal world views.

The central thesis of this book is that the biblical world view is not a blend of the Western and primal world views. Rather, the biblical world view is a third way that affirms the validity of some assumptions from each world view. This world view profoundly affects the way we think about the role of development work in Christian missions.

The book transforms both world views by enabling us to see God working redemptively through the normal processes of creation. The first section of the book addresses the importance of understanding the assumptions we make about reality.

This section shows how Paul's problem in Lystra is repeated throughout the world. Christian missionaries and development practitioners do a variety of tasks to redeem creation in the name of Christ. While they go about their tasks, they must provide an interpretation of that work to communicate how it contributes to the redemptive work of Christ. Otherwise, the Christians and their hosts will interpret the work according to the assumptions of their world views, neglecting or misinterpreting the place of *shalom* in their work.

The second section of the book suggests how the particular disciplines of development contribute to the redemptive work of Christ. The central point of these chapters is that the various pursuits of development—such as education, economics, ecology and medicine—are intrinsically valuable to our participation in Christ's redemptive work in creation. These chapters go beyond the commonly held idea that these pursuits are valuable if we flavor them with Christian values. The chapters affirm the importance of these values, but they also stress that values are not enough. We need to interpret these disciplines so they participate in the redemptive ministry of Christ by bringing *shalom* to creation.

The final section of the book brings closure by proposing ways of evaluating and communicating the presence of shalom as a symbol of God's redemptive work in a particular culture and throughout creation. The message of this section is that God transforms ordinary elements of creation to bear witness to his presence in a particular culture.

ONE

Shalom:
The bridge between
development and evangelism

. . . yet my unfailing love for you will not be shaken
nor my covenant of peace be removed . . .
Isaiah 54:10

"The Spirit of the Lord is on me,
because he has anointed me
to preach good news to the poor.
He has sent me to proclaim freedom for the prisoners
and recovery of sight for the blind,
to release the oppressed,
to proclaim the year of the Lord's favor."
Luke 4:18-19

For he himself is our peace,
who has made the two one . . .
his purpose was to create in himself
one new man out of two, thus making peace.
Ephesians 2:14-15

MOST CHRISTIAN MISSIONS and Christian development agencies have struggled with defining the relationship between development and evangelism. Often, the problem is discerning whether development has, or should have, an evangelistic impact.

Western cultures, particularly, see development and evangelism as separate enterprises—development is not necessarily evangelistic. The thinking is that evangelism addresses spiritual needs while development addresses physical needs.

5

The separation of evangelism from development creates a gap in Christian missions that is causing increasing dissatisfaction among development agencies.

Some agencies ask: If development does not have an evangelistic impact, what is its purpose? Can we bridge the gap between development and evangelism, or should development become the second item on the agenda of Christian missions? Is development a valid need for Christians to meet? Can it be met after the world is evangelized?

Other agencies have a commitment to development, and believe development has an evangelistic impact. The questions these agencies ask include: How is the evangelistic impact of development expressed? Does the evangelistic impact of development speak for itself, or does development prove the worth of the spoken, evangelistic word?

The following situations depict some efforts made by Christian missions to bridge the gap between evangelism and development.

Efforts to bridge the gap

A bus crashed in an Islamic village in the Sahel. Dozens of people were injured, and the village hospital did not have adequate medical supplies to care for them.

A Christian mission had several medical projects in the village. It provided personnel, food, clothing and medical supplies to treat the victims of the crash. The team members of the mission expressed a variety of views on the relationship between evangelism and development as they prepared their relief aid. One team member, who valued relief and development efforts because they led to opportunities for evangelism, wanted to include Scripture verses in the donated materials. Providing relief materials without including a spiritual message proved unsatisfactory to him.

Another team member, for a variety of reasons, was uncomfortable with including the Scripture verses in the relief supplies. He believed the relief and development efforts were intrinsically valid expressions of Christian spirituality. He saw relief and development as parallel expressions of Christian ministry. He had no trouble feeding the hungry, healing the sick or empowering the impoverished when opportunities for evangelism were not possible.

This team member also believed providing the Scriptures would injure the commitment the mission made to the government not to proselytize. "Providing the Scriptures is an act of evangelism or proselytism," he protested, "we cannot do it. We registered in this country as a humanitarian Christian organization. If we include Scripture verses with anything we give to the Islamic community, we are guilty of violating our trust with the community and the government. The integrity of Christ in this country depends on our honoring that agreement."

"How much risk is there in letting the people know the source of their blessings?" asked the team member who raised the issue. "The people know we are Christians, and they respect us as people called by God to work in this village. The Scripture verses are not going to tell them what they do not already know. Our work and presence in this community already communicate the redemptive message of Christ. God does not need a return address on his blessings."

A third team member believed relief and development efforts should follow evangelism. He thought that the community would not respond to relief and development efforts by Christians because the people could not appreciate Christian values unless they knew Christ. Until then, such efforts would fall on deaf ears or blind eyes. He concluded that relief and development work should be done only where Christians could openly preach the gospel.

What is unique about Christian development?

In another African village, members of a Western[1] Christian development agency dug a well. They then analyzed the water and found a high concentration of phosphates in it. Since the cost of purifying the water was more than the village or the agency could afford, both faced a difficult problem. What would they do about the contaminated well? Was there a spiritual solution to this physical problem?

The Christians who built the well accepted the limitations of economics and science, and advised the people in the community not to drink the water. They instructed the people to use the well water only for livestock and irrigation. They further explained how phosphates are likely to cause health problems and birth defects.

The villagers approached the problem differently. They called the village shaman to exorcise spirits from the well. Although the villagers had developed considerable respect for the Christian agency personnel, their approach to solving the problem was one of the many ways in which the villagers differed from the missionaries. The villagers reasoned, "If there are phosphates in the well, they cannot just happen to be there. The spirits must be causing the phosphates to be in the well. If we appease the spirits," the villagers reasoned, "the phosphates would go away."

The village shaman led the community in a ceremony to purify the water. The ceremony included dancing, chanting, singing, an animal sacrifice, and throwing burning incense into the well. After the ceremony, the concentration of phosphates in the water remained unchanged.

Apparently, the spirits, for whatever reason, were unwilling or unable to purify the well.

When the Christians gathered for a Bible study, a new team member expressed his feelings of discontentment about the villagers performing a ceremony to purify the well. He believed there was something more *spiritual* about the villagers' attempt to solve the problem. "What are we communicating about the spirituality of Christianity," he asked the other team members, "when we build a well, and the non-Christians perform a religious ceremony to purify it?"

"That is a deep issue," the team leader responded with an intended pun. "Are you suggesting that Christians should perform a ceremony to purify the well?"

The new member responded, "Our problem is that our wells say nothing about our spirituality. We accepted the contamination as a scientific or physical limitation. It was beyond our control, but is it beyond God's control? What are we communicating about God when we do not invoke his power to bless our work? Does God have the power to remove the phosphates from the well? Why don't we invoke the power of God as the shaman attempted to invoke the power of the spirits?"

"We are praying for God's blessing on our ministry," another team member replied, "and the community is aware of our spirituality. Still, we must accept contaminated wells—along with hunger, illness and death—as facts of life in a fallen world. These results of a fallen creation grieve God much more than they grieve us."

"My problem," the new team member continued, "is that we are making so little effort to express the spirituality of our work. I'm not suggesting that we perform a Christian ceremony to purify the wells; maybe we should. But my problem is determining if we are any different from non-Christian agencies. The wells they dig are no different from the ones we dig. This leaves us with the question: 'What is unique about Christian development?'"

"Our dilemma," the team leader interjected, "is that we are communicating a relationship with a sovereign God in a physical environment that is degenerating. Our role in this relationship is a role of reconciliation. We are working toward reconciling to God a creation that is degenerating from the general and particular effects of sin. In this regard, wells, the media of our work, are not unique. Yet our message differs from other agencies. We are digging wells to participate in the redemptive ministry of Christ.

"This ministry of reconciliation is progressive," she continued. "It is already happening, but is *not yet* realized in its fullness. The well is a result of a fallen creation.

"Our temptation in this ministry is to emulate the methods of the shaman. He attempts to facilitate change through a form of magic. When he led the ceremony, the shaman expected the behavior of the people in the community to influence the spirits to purify the well. If he had been successful in influencing the spirits to purify the well, he would have been a power broker.

"In contrast to the shaman, we are not power brokers; we are peacemakers. We do not express the redemptive power of God through a stronger form of magic, a form of magic that gives us power over the spirits and the community. Rather, we express God's redemptive power through the covenant of peace that God has made with creation. The power of the gospel is not stronger than the shaman's power; it is of a different nature."

"Is this *already-not yet* approach to Christian ministry one that we can build an evangelism strategy on?" the new member asked.

"Yes," the team leader replied, "it has to be. Otherwise, we would create a dichotomy that separates evangelism from development, or the physical dimension of creation. This separation would weaken the greatest strength of this society—its integration of what Westerners categorize as physical and spiritual issues. Our calling is not to impose a dichotomy on the culture that separates the Christian message from our work. Our calling is to reveal the redemptive work of Christ within the culture.

"Wells, by regenerating the deteriorating environment, witness to God's redemptive work in this culture. Separating the physical and spiritual aspects of redemption is not Good News to these people or anyone else. We cannot separate our media from our message of reconciliation and redemption."

Communicating redemption cross-culturally

In a third village, Jama was a recent convert from Islam to Christianity. Since his conversion, his wife, Anab, had been unable to get pregnant. She and her Muslim sisters were convinced that her infertility was a curse from Allah.

Jama was not sure what to think. He did not believe his wife was cursed, but he had trouble understanding exactly how his new faith addressed his wife's infertility. He and Anab had four children, and she had no trouble getting pregnant until he became a Christian. "Do Christians have signs, symbols or sacrifices to facilitate pregnancies?" he wondered. His question hinted at his need to transform the cultural symbols of fertility to communicate meaning in Christianity.

Jama talked to the Christians about his wife's infertility, and they told him how fertility decreases as women get older. Since he and his wife wanted to have a fifth child, the Christians committed themselves to praying for Anab to get pregnant. Jama appreciated the prayer, but it seemed parenthetical to the problem. The Christians appeared to accept Anab's infertility as a result of her natural aging process. They did not communicate confidence in their prayers for Anab to get pregnant

The lack of confidence in the prayers puzzled Jama. "How does the God of the Christians answer prayers?" he wondered. "Do the missionaries really expect that God will intervene in nature to enable Anab to get pregnant?"

Meanwhile, Anab visited a local sheikh, an Islamic spiritual leader, who insisted on seeing her husband. The sheikh believed that Jama's conversion brought a curse on the family. Anab's infertility was only the first of many misfortunes the sheikh expected to result from the curse. The extended family would experience many problems because of Jama's conversion. The family's only hope to reverse the curse was to have Jama make a sacrifice to Allah. Otherwise, Jama would have to be ostracized from the family.

Jama returned to the missionaries and asked: "What more can be done about my wife's infertility? If Anab becomes pregnant, her anxiety—at least for a time—will be solved."

The missionaries sent Jama to a Christian medical doctor who listened empathetically, but offered little help. The doctor recommended that Anab take fertility pills, but Jama flatly rejected the idea. Anab would never take pills to get pregnant. She only knew about taking pills to prevent pregnancy, an idea she and her sisters staunchly resisted. She also heard that the hospital staff gave immunizations to women and children. The staff said the immunizations would prevent disease, but the women in the village believed the injections were causing infertility.

Jama anticipated his wife asking, "Why would the foreign doctor give pills to cause pregnancy when he also gives them to prevent pregnancy?" Besides, the sheikh said Anab's infertility was the result of a curse, something that only Allah could reverse.

When Jama came home from the visit, he noticed an ostrich egg, the local symbol of fertility, on the roof of his house. Anab, realizing that her husband would not visit the sheikh, chose another means of solving her infertility problem. The belief was that ostrich eggs, while not having the power of a sacrifice to Allah, helped infertile women get pregnant. Jama made another visit to the missionaries and asked them, "Does the ostrich egg on the roof of my house make a statement that Christians can accept?"

The initial consensus of the missionaries was not to affirm the use of the ostrich egg. They felt the egg represented an unhealthy compromise between the spiritual convictions of Jama and those of Anab. If Jama acquiesced to placing the egg on the roof of his house, he may be vulnerable to submitting to the spiritual authority of the Islamic community.

Jama was not fully convinced that the missionaries understood his situation. He believed the ostrich egg was a cultural rather than a religious symbol. "Yes," he granted, "the egg represents power, but it is not the spiritual power of Islam. It is the power of fertility, a generic power that exists in every culture.

"The ostrich egg is like jewelry," Jama continued. "People do not believe jewelry has power, but they wear it to symbolize particular powers. The egg, likewise, represents the power of fertility. Why can't the egg symbolize God's power to bring fertility to my family in a culturally relevant way?"

"Jama, what statement does the egg make to the community about your faith?" one missionary asked. While Jama was thinking about his answer, another person mentioned that God works through culturally relevant media. This person suggested, "The egg is a culturally relevant symbol of fertility. If Jama can interpret the symbolism of the egg to be meaningful in his Christian faith, it should be displayed."

That answer did not satisfy the missionary who asked the question. He wondered how the community could be evangelized if Jama did not make a cleaner break with either Islam or the culture.

Jama was not comfortable continuing the conversation about symbols; he wanted to get to the root of the problem. He asked about the spirituality of the fertility pills that were recommended to him. "What do they say about the power of God?"

One missionary mentioned that fertility pills solve a physical, not a spiritual, problem. Yet he affirmed they could be used by God to fulfill his will, and would become spiritual when administered with prayer. The missionary responded, "That is the holistic nature of our mission. Through prayer, we spiritually anoint the physical side of our ministry."

The distinctions between the physical and spiritual were making little sense to Jama. "If you did not prayerfully anoint the medicine," he asked, "would it still be effective? How do you make distinctions between physical and spiritual problems?"

The ensuing discussion raised several answers that were both complementary and contradictory. Most of the answers focused on development and evangelism; the missionaries agreed that development addressed physical problems while evangelism addressed spiritual ones. Physical problems include health, agriculture, education and economics. Spiritual problems, in contrast, include, among other things, salvation, spiritual growth, and forgiveness.

By spiritually anointing the medicine, we make an evangelistic statement. We affirm our commitment to God and his commitment to us. The effectiveness of the medicine probably would be the same with or without prayer, but we need the prayer to communicate the spiritual message of our work. We believe God is the source of healing, and we pray to acknowledge and communicate that belief. He heals whether or not we acknowledge his role in healing. Evangelism is acknowledging his role.

Jama still was not satisfied that there was a solution to his problem. He believed the holistic Christian development practitioners understood his problem, but their answers made distinctions and assumptions he did not make. The distinction between the physical and spiritual natures of the problem, and the evangelistic implications of the solutions, for example, were difficult for Jama to separate. For the holistic Christian development practitioners, the spiritual and evangelistic implications of the problem seemed synonymous.

It seemed to Jama that in the name of holism the missionaries related the physical and spiritual natures of the problem, but still saw them as separate dimensions of reality. For Jama, though, the nature of his wife's infertility could not be divided; it was intrinsically spiritual.

Evangelism, for Jama, was a separate issue. Before the evangelistic implications of the solutions could be addressed, the infertility problem had to be solved. Jama wanted to realize God's power in enabling Anab to get pregnant. For him, the spirituality of the problem and the evangelistic implications of the solutions, while not dichotomous, were separate. Evangelism was not the spiritual dimension of the problem, but it was an implication of the problem that would follow the solution.

Jama asked the missionaries, "In what ways is God's power realized in addressing my wife's infertility? The physical and spiritual aspects of my problem seem to be on opposite sides of a river. Development addresses one side of the river and evangelism addresses the other. You believe your ministry is comprehensive, or holistic, because it addresses both sides of the river. But is there a bridge that symbolizes the spirituality of Christian missions by unifying these separate aspects of ministry?"

Jama's question raised important issues related to holism: Is the comprehensive approach to ministry really holistic, or does holism imply a greater integration of the physical and spiritual elements in the redemptive work of Christ? Does holism change the nature of development by making it holy?

The nature of the problem

The central problem in each of the preceding situations, as Figure

Figure 1.1   The relationship of high religion, folk religion and science[2]

Level	Focus	Questions concerning . . .
High/ Orthodox Religion	Truth	• Ultimate origins and destiny • Meaning and purpose in life
Low/Folk Religion (e.g., animism)	Power	• Well-being: diseases, famine, drought • Guidance: fear, uncertainty of the future • Success, failure • Peace: dealing with spirit world and spirit possession
Science	Control	• Control over nature by technology • Hostile world and difficulties • Social harmony: social conflict, wars, rivalries, feuds

1.1 above illustrates, is an understanding of the relationship between religious truth, religious power, and science. Major world religions, such as Christianity and Islam, as expressed in their higher forms, focus on truth and raise questions about the ultimate meaning and purpose of life. Animism and the folk expressions of major religions focus on power. They deal with health, well-being, guidance, success and failure.

The ultimate issue in animism and folk religions is being at peace with the spirit world. In folk beliefs, truth, in the ultimate sense of expressing meaning and purpose, becomes incidental to power. Power, not truth, protects people from the calamities that threaten their physical safety, their economic welfare and spiritual well-being.

The concern of science, in contrast to orthodox and folk religions, is control. It "is not only a way of knowing and a way of viewing the world; it is also a way of doing, a way of controlling nature."[3] It focuses on "observing the relationships between events, proposing explanations for these relationships, and controlling the relationships to achieve a foreseeable outcome."[4]

From a modern, Western perspective, science and the orthodox expressions of Christianity have had a somewhat compatible existence. Religion serves as a basis for morality, purpose and meaning in the lives of individuals and society, while science attempts to solve the physical problems of life.

The problem we face in modern, Western society is religion's inability to maintain its role of giving meaning to life in the face of science and technology. We are developing an "unqualified reliance on technology."[5] This reliance on technology frequently prevents us from seeing how God expresses his redemptive work through science and technology. It leads us to see science and technology as autonomous from God. Scientific and technological innovations have largely become ends in themselves. We no longer interpret what they mean to us in the context of our faith.

For Christians with a non-Western world view, where technology has not been so invasive, God's power is esteemed to deliver them from the spiritual and physical threats to their well-being. This esteem for God's power is the pulse of people who embrace non-Western, or primal, world views. They esteem God not only for providing people with an ultimate purpose and meaning in life, but also because he provides for their every need.

In fact, God's provision for their daily needs is more central to their faith than his providing an ultimate meaning for their lives. When they cannot find adequate food, shelter, or medical care, a faith that focuses on their ultimate purposes in life is irrelevant. They need the guidance, peace and security that come with the provision for their daily sustenance.

The differences between primal and modern world views became apparent in the three anecdotes mentioned earlier in this chapter. In applying Figure 1.1 to the efforts of purifying the well, evangelizing the community, or solving Anab's infertility problem, the indigenous people in each situation focused on the power of their faith to facilitate change. Jama wanted to understand how the power of God, as known by Christians, addressed his wife's infertility. The village shaman attempted to appease the spirits to invoke their power to purify the well. For each of them, the power of their religious experience was like electricity going through electrical appliances: we value electricity for its ability to run appliances.

In contrast, the missionaries focused on what they saw as the ultimate meaning and purpose of their faith. The mission leader who advocated peace as the symbol of the reconciliation and redemption of Christian missions accepted the limits of science and focused on communicating God's covenant of peace within the fallen creation. The missionaries who addressed Jama's problem also accepted the limits of science. Yet they focused on evangelism as the ultimate purpose of their work.

Evangelism was the ultimate purpose of the missionary who wanted to include Scripture passages with relief supplies, and he wanted to use science to achieve that end. He knew a relationship existed between the number of tracts he distributed and the number of converts he could expect in a particular community, and he wanted to apply that knowledge to his particular situation. He attempted to gain some control over the evangelistic impact of his relief efforts by adding the tracts.

Our concern with this missionary's approach is not with the validity of his knowledge, but with its application. Undoubtedly he was correct in believing a relationship existed between distributing tracts and gaining converts. But he faced legal and philosophical problems.

On the one hand, he was dealing with the legal implications of distributing the tracts in a community that did not make a distinction between evangelism and proselytism, and forbade both activities.

On the other hand, he worked with a mission that was philosophically opposed to separating development from evangelism. The other members of his team saw their work as holistic, not comprehensive or dualistic. They were firm believers in personal evangelism, and felt that any evangelistic efforts in the community had to be done through personal relationships. They felt the tracts would impede the relationships they were building with the people in the community.

The spiritual assumptions of the missionaries and the indigenous people clashed because the missionaries, unlike the indigenous people, separated God from creation. The meaning the missionaries found in their faith was not necessarily connected to the environment in which they lived. Instead, they based their relationship with God on a hope of salvation that transcended physical circumstances. The question for them was finding how they could use the circumstances to bring people in relationship to the ultimate truth and meaning in life that God provides.

The indigenous people could not separate God from their surroundings. They believed God gives life to everything in the seen and unseen realms. Their perception of God's power in the environment is somewhat analogous to electricity working in appliances. Electricity cannot be seen, but its presence is evident when an appliance is operating.

Just as people in some cultures cannot envision electricity apart from the wires and appliances through which it is conducted, people in primal cultures do not envision the power of God apart from the objects to which God gives life and power. In primal cultures, God's power is not abstract, but is apparent in the physical objects that house it; the power of God cannot be homeless.

To use a different aspect of the electricity analogy, electricity, like the power of God, cannot be seen but it can be felt. If people from a primal culture believe the power of God is in a particular object, they would, in all likelihood, feel something if they touch the object. If the power in the object is strong enough, the people could get a shock.

An aspect of this concept of God's power residing in physical objects has been integrated into Western culture in an amusing way.

Many universities have traditions of "academic chairs." In a seminary I attended, a distinguished professor of theology received the "Andrew Mutch Chair of Systematic Theology."

I understand this tradition came to Europe from the Islamic cultures during the Crusades. The originators of the tradition would have understood that the power that Andrew Mutch received from God was physically present in the actual chair in which Andrew Mutch sat. If the originators of the tradition visited the professor who currently occupies the chair, they would expect to see Andrew Mutch's original chair. Otherwise, the divine power that enabled Andrew Mutch to be an effective teacher was lost. Chairs that Andrew Mutch did not sit in could not possibly contain his power.

The missionaries in the previous situations did not grasp the tangible nature of God's power. Therefore, they attempted to make the connection between their faith and their work by integrating what they believed to be physical and spiritual components. They had medical, well-drilling and relief projects to meet physical needs, and evangelistic efforts to meet spiritual needs. To the extent that their work was integrated, they called it holistic, implying they were making their work a holy service, or offering, to God.

Yet they did not solve the problem of portraying God's participation in their work as anything but an unexpected miraculous or mystical event. This left the people questioning whether the holistic nature of their work was exceptional or normal. In this respect, their work appeared comprehensive because it incorporated the spiritual and physical aspects of life. But it fell short of communicating a holistic nature in the work. Holistic ministry is not synonymous with comprehensive ministry.

Christian ministry is holistic, not comprehensive

The central theme of this monograph is the intrinsic relationship between evangelism and development. This relationship exists because Christ's redemptive work includes the entire creation, things seen and unseen. In this sense, redemption is defined as restoring the elements of creation to fulfill the purposes for which God created them.

Holism does not see non-human life or inanimate matter participating in salvation as people participate in it, but it seeks to restore the harmony of creation that reflects the glory of God. To this extent, distinctions between evangelism and development, or the physical and spiritual aspects of creation, are detrimental to our understanding and fulfilling the call of Christians to ministry. The visible, physical aspects of creation as well as the invisible, spiritual aspects must be harmonized to support the abundant life we have in Christ.

Luke 4:18-19, the passage Jesus used to inaugurate his ministry, illustrates the holistic nature of Christian ministry. In it, Jesus affirms that the poor will hear the Good News, the prisoners will be freed, the blind will see, the oppressed will be liberated, and he proclaims Jubilee, the year of the Lord's favor. The society of Israel will be renewed. There will be no more waiting; the Good News of the kingdom of God has arrived.

The problem we have in understanding the nature of Jesus' ministry, and in fulfilling his mandate, is making a relationship between preaching, advocating justice and ministering to the poor, naked, sick, hungry, and oppressed. Do we advocate justice and minister to the poor, naked, sick, hungry, and oppressed because it gives us the opportunity to preach the Good News to them? Or is advocating justice and ministering to the poor, sick, naked, hungry, and oppressed, in itself, good news? Holism affirms that ministering to the poor, sick, naked, hungry, and oppressed and preaching the message of eternal salvation is Good News.

A major reason why we have trouble connecting evangelism and development is our lack of a term to communicate the connection. Even if we agree that development participates in the redemptive nature of Christian ministry, we have not fully defined what we mean when we say so.

Evangelism clearly states the Good News of Jesus Christ is salvation to all who believe. Development, on the other hand, attempts to relieve the vulnerability to pain and suffering that people experience when they live in deteriorating conditions.

However, the biblical concepts of development and evangelism are not separate. The Greek words commonly used for healing—*soteria* and *sozo*, for example—also mean salvation. These words blur the distinction we tend to make as we think of healing and salvation as physical or spiritual ministries. Other biblical concepts, such as *koinonia*, or fellowship, also have physical and spiritual connotations.

Shalom is the key to understanding holism

Therefore, in light of only a few biblical teachings, the need for a term to communicate the connection between development and evangelism becomes apparent. That word is *shalom*.[6]

Generally translated *peace*, the concept of *shalom* means more than the mere absence of war, our common definition of peace.[7] Instead, *shalom* is a concept that communicates the sense of "human welfare, health and well-being, in both spiritual and material aspects."[8] *Shalom* is a way of life that characterizes the covenant relationship between God and his people. Malachi declares this covenant to be one of "life and *shalom*" (Mal. 2:5).

We frequently think of the covenant between God and his people as a covenant of salvation, yet salvation is but one aspect of *shalom*. *Shalom* also defines the state of wholeness and holiness possessed by individuals and communities as they become part of the greater community of faith.

"[*Shalom*] describes the condition of well-being resulting from the sound relationships among people and between people and God."[9] "It includes social justice: the protection of widows, orphans, and society's dependents; the struggle against exploitation and oppression; the protection of life and property."[10]

Shalom is the "expression of harmony intended by God."[11] Robert McAfee Brown defined the term as "shockingly materialistic."[12] While it goes beyond the absence of war, it also transcends the sense of personal peace that Christians use to spiritualize the term. "It has to do," wrote Brown, "with the state of one's belly, whether it is full or empty, whether it is a source of health or disease; it has to do with having adequate shelter; it has to do with security that is physical as well as spiritual."[13] "Nature itself is included in *shalom*."[14] "From the disruption of *shalom* in the Garden of Eden to its total renewal in the new Jerusalem, the object of all God's work is the recovery of *shalom* in his creation."[15]

A concept of development that is both Christian and holistic emphasizes revealing God's presence and empowering people to experience the principles of the kingdom that *shalom* embodies. Holistic Christian development, characterized by *shalom*, recognizes that the gospel has present and future tenses. We look forward to the day when the kingdom of God will be revealed in its fullness. Yet we also have the present hope that the kingdom of God is with us and brings peace to our present life situations.

Because of the present and future hope of the gospel, holism affirms that poverty, oppression and injustice are not incidental to revealing the redemptive nature of the gospel. Rather, the Good News of Christ cannot be revealed without speaking to these issues. To use the famous concept of Marshall McLuhan, the medium is the message. *Shalom*, as it addresses poverty, oppression and injustice, is the medium that comprises the liberating message of a development approach that is both Christian and holistic.

Shalom bridges the gap between development and evangelism by its concern for truth, power and control. It does not see these things as contradictory or competitive, but sees their roles redemptively. God works to bring these aspects of high religion, folk religion and science together within *shalom*. It is a comprehensive term that defies the categories within which we want to place it. As Ulrich Mauser writes: "The neat separation of a 'secular' from a 'sacred' domain is, after all, of very modern vintage, and one may suspect the ancient Israelites would not have comprehended it."[16] Through *shalom*, truth, power and control have a place in making known the covenant that reconciles creation to the Creator.

NOTES

1. The words "modern" and "Western" are used interchangeably throughout this book. They refer "to a state of mind, more than a geographical location, that includes the individualism, scientism, social evolution, egalitarianism, and self-actualization referred to in modern thought" (*Pastoral Counseling Across Cultures*, David W. Augsburger [Philadelphia: Westminster Press, 1986], p. 15).

2. Based on a chart found in *Phenomenology and Institutions of Folk Religions*, Paul G. Hiebert (Pasadena: Fuller Theological Seminary, 1990), p. 21.

3. Ian G. Barbour, *Science and Secularity: The Ethics of Technology* (New York: Harper and Row, 1970), p. 59.

4. David Burns, personal correspondence, January 1992.

5. Barbour, p. 67.

6. In this book, *shalom* is defined as "the harmony God intended for creation." In the Greek New Testament *shalom* is translated *eirene*; in English it is translated "peace." Neither *eirene* nor "peace" communicate the concept of harmony in creation as well as *shalom*. I regret how the word has become associated with Zionism, but I have chosen to use it despite this use.

7. *Shalom*, in fact, does not necessarily mean the absence of war.

8. Marlin E. Miller, "The Gospel of Peace," *Mission and Peace Witness*, Robert L. Ramseyer, ed. (Scottdale: Herald Press, 1978), p. 30.

9. Ibid.

10. Sjouke Voolstra, "The Search for a Biblical Peace Testimony," *Mission and Peace Witness*, Robert L. Ramseyer, ed. (Scottdale: Herald Press, 1978), p. 30.

11. Bernard Haring, *The Healing Power of Peace and Non-Violence* (Maryknoll: Paulist Press, 1986), p. 32.

12. Robert McAfee Brown, *Making Peace in the Global Village* (Philadelphia: The Westminster Press, 1981), p. 14.

13. Ibid.

14. Voolstra, p. 30.

15. James E. Metzler, "Shalom is the Mission," *Mission and Peace Witness*, Robert L. Ramseyer, ed. (Scottdale: Herald Press, 1978), p. 40.

16. Ulrich Mauser, *The Gospel of Peace* (Louisville: Westminster/John Knox Press, 1992), p. 17.

TWO

World views:
Transforming our perceptions

Then the sailors said to each other,
"Come, let us cast lots to find out
who is responsible for this calamity."
They cast lots and the lot fell on Jonah.
Jonah 1:7

For God was pleased to have all his fullness dwell in him,
and through him to reconcile to himself all things,
whether things on earth or things in heaven,
by making peace through his blood, shed on the cross.
Colossians 1:19-20

PEOPLE WHO LIVE in different cultures have different ways of organizing their perceptions of the world.

People from Western cultures are likely to organize the world by separating its physical aspects from its spiritual aspects. This separation creates a dichotomy between the physical and spiritual dimensions of reality.

People from non-Western cultures, such as Africans, perceive a constant interaction between the physical and spiritual aspects of creation. They believe Christian theology splits "humans into body and soul, and to preach the salvation of the soul. Africa could never accept this mutilation of the human being."[1]

The impact of differing world views

I realized the impact of the differences between Western and primal cultures when I taught in an African culture. One day, one of my students mentioned that his father had broken his leg. Our world views caused us to have different understandings of why that misfortune happened.

"How did that happen?" I asked the student.

"A donkey kicked him," came the reply.

"It must have been a swift kick," I responded, with the satisfaction that the kick adequately explained the misfortune.

"The people in the village are trying to learn why it happened," the student continued.

At this point, I realized the student and I were making different assumptions. I classified the broken leg as a misfortune, and believed the cause of the broken leg was accidental. As far as I was concerned, the student's father got too close to a donkey, and the donkey kicked him. While I had trouble believing the kick was strong enough to break a leg, I saw the problem in terms of cause-and-effect within the physical realm. I did not believe there was more to the story.

But there was more to the story. The student and his family believed the father was a victim of spiritual powers. They did not believe, as I did, that the donkey randomly kicked the man. They were confident that there was a reason for the donkey kicking the man at that particular time. The man had walked behind the donkey many times before and the donkey had not kicked him. They concluded that the timing of this kick was not coincidental. Therefore, the donkey was not to blame for the misfortune; he was merely an instrument of a higher power.

In their world view, the relationship between the spiritual realm and the physical realm adequately explained the incident. Blaming the donkey was simply settling for the intermediate cause of the event. In the minds of the villagers, the central question was, "Who caused the donkey to kick at the particular moment when the man was behind the donkey?"

The villagers wanted to learn the root cause of the misfortune. They saw the world as the arena in which spiritual forces interact with the physical to bring fortune and misfortune on people. To understand the cause of this misfortune, the villagers had to understand who cursed the father or used witchcraft on him. Was the power that caused the donkey to kick the man an angry ancestor, or an enemy of the family or clan? Or did someone pay a sorcerer to curse the father or the family?

Finding the answer to these questions required that the family consult sorcerers or other people with spiritual discernment. Such people would, in turn, communicate with the spirits or the ancestors. These people also could manipulate charms, mana or other impersonal powers to find the ultimate cause of the problem.

None of these methods of spiritual discernment fit into my world view. As a Christian with a modern, Western world view, I saw the event

Figure 2.1   One view of the world

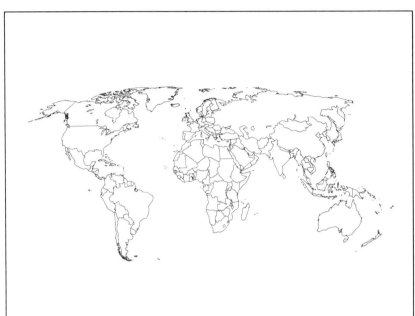

Figure 2.2   Another view of the world

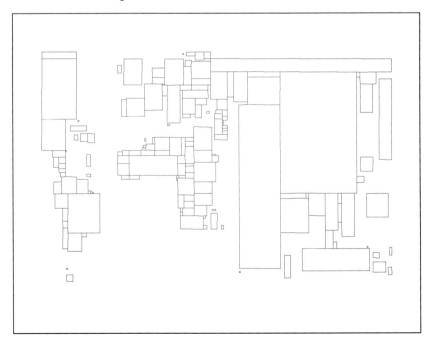

as unfortunate, but could not offer an explanation that would satisfy the student or his family. Why do bad things happen to good people? Is misfortune caused by sorcery? Does it satisfy us to believe that human carelessness, which causes humankind so much grief, is random or unprovoked? These problems separate one world view from another.

The roles of world views in our lives

World views are like maps: they provide us with a theme for organizing our perceptions of the world.

Figures 2.1 and 2.2 on page 23 contain two maps that show different ways of picturing our environments. Since each map gives us a different view of how the world is arranged, each also gives us a different basis for making decisions, evaluations and judgments.

The first map assumes that land formations are important. The second map, in organizing countries by the sizes of their human populations, assumes that land formations are unimportant.

The validity of each map depends on the decisions we are making. For people who are traveling, the top map is important. Land formations give us an idea of how far apart particular countries are. The bottom map assumes that human population has no relationship to land formations. The countries with the largest populations are not necessarily those with the largest number of square kilometers.

If we want to see the world in terms of human population, the map in Figure 2.2 is more useful than the map in Figure 2.1. The map in Figure 2.1 will actually mislead us.

In making decisions regarding population problems, such as infant mortality, Figure 2.2 is also more useful. It shows that countries such as India, Bangladesh, Nigeria, Indonesia and China have large human populations. So these countries are more likely to have higher numbers of infant deaths, and possibly a higher infant mortality rate. This data is not obvious in Figure 2.1. Nigeria, Bangladesh and Indonesia, particularly, have small areas of land in relation to the sizes of their population.

World views, like maps, influence many decisions in our lives. The missionaries mentioned in chapter one confronted different world views in addressing the problems of the contaminated wells, Anab's infertility, and the evangelistic impact of their relief and development work. Our ability to see that development participates in the redemptive work of Christ, and that *shalom* is the symbol that connects development and evangelism, depends on our world view. I could not comprehend my student's concern for *who* caused his father's misfortune because we had different world views, or maps of reality.

Figure 2.3   Western world view   Figure 2.4   Primal world view

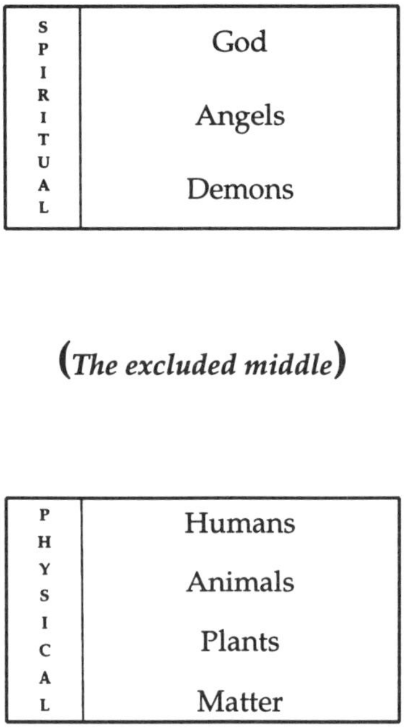

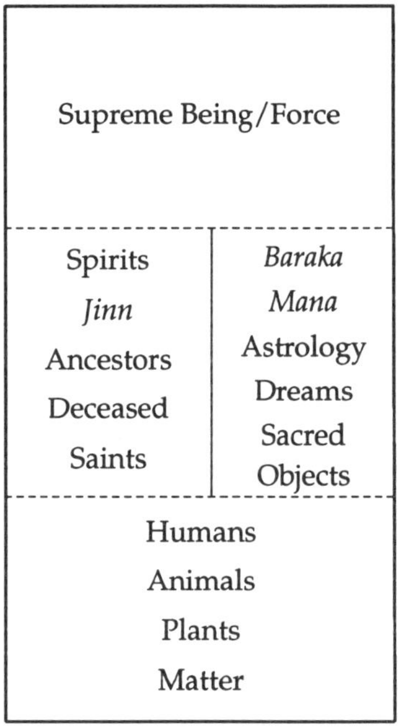

S P I R I T U A L	God Angels Demons

(*The excluded middle*)

P H Y S I C A L	Humans Animals Plants Matter

Supreme Being/Force

Spirits *Jinn* Ancestors Deceased Saints	*Baraka* *Mana* Astrology Dreams Sacred Objects

Humans Animals Plants Matter

Figures 2.3 and 2.4 above illustrate the two separate maps of reality with which the student and I made our assumptions.[2] He believed the spiritual beings or spiritual forces in Figure 2.4 caused the donkey to kick his father. My view of reality prevented me from affirming this assumption. I did not make a connection between the physical and spiritual realms. I based my assumption on seeing the physical realm as separate from the spiritual realm. In my view, the donkey acted on its own initiative.

The differing assumptions in Figures 2.3 and 2.4 commonly affect Christian missions. They do not account for every world view operating in other cultures around the world, but they represent broad classifications. When Christians from a Western culture go to a non-Western culture, they are likely to import the Western world view in Figure 2.3 and confront the primal world view in Figure 2.4.

Characteristics of primal world views

Primal world views organize the world around relationships of power between physical and spiritual forces. In religions that develop within primal world views, such as folk expressions of major world religions and African traditional religions, the supreme deities are distant: relating to them is not so important. The stories of most primal religions show that the supreme deities were closer to the earth at one time, but they left for a variety of reasons. In some cultures, the people believe they had offended the supreme deities, who then became angry and withdrew their presence from the earth. In other cultures, someone had poked the supreme deities with a spear or hit them with a club, and the deities decided heaven was safer than earth.

Relationships with the lesser spiritual beings and spiritual forces provide the spiritual power of primal religions. "In short, there is a continuous exchange going on between the visible and the invisible worlds."[3]

These forces and beings, which comprise "the middle" of primal cultures, include, among other entities, local gods, goddesses, spirits, ancestors, and deceased saints. The spiritual forces include *mana*, *baraka*, astrology, charms, amulets, and various forms of magic. These forces normally interact with human and non-human life, and with inanimate matter. The media of this interaction include, but are not limited to, prayers, spells, curses, dreams, visions, sacrifices, rituals and ceremonies.

Anthropologists and missiologists—Paul Hiebert in particular— categorize these spirits and impersonal forces as *the excluded middle.*[4] They are considered excluded, as Figure 2.3 shows, because they do not fit into the world views of the modern, Western missiologists who work in primal cultures. They are part of the unseen reality of the primal cultures that modern cultures marginalize or remove.

People appease and manipulate the spirits of the excluded middle to bring healing and health, prosperity, security, or meaning to life. When good things happen, people believe that the spirits are responding favorably to prayers, rites, rituals and any other forms of worship.

Natural or unexplained causes of illness, death or misfortune are not foreign to primal world views. Yet they are not the first place people with primal world views look when they attempt to understand *why* something happened. Like the family that wanted to know *who* caused the donkey to kick the man, people with primal world views want to know who causes misfortunes. For example, the crew on the ship that the prophet Jonah boarded for Tarshish wanted to know who caused the storm that jeopardized their safety. After casting lots, they learned that Jonah was responsible (Jonah 1:7).

The question in understanding events from the perspective of primal world views does not seek an answer that conforms to the logic of cause-and-effect that is characteristic of problem-solving in modern world views. David Burnett eloquently explains this characteristic of the primal world view in the following dialogue:

Tribesman: This man is sick because someone worked sorcery against him.

White Doctor: This man is sick from malaria because he was bitten by an infected mosquito!

Tribesman: Yes, he was bitten by a mosquito—but *who* sent the mosquito?[5]

Characteristics of the modern theistic world view

The modern theistic world view, similar to the primal world view, sees the influence of God on all human enterprises. Yet unlike people with a primal world view, people who hold a modern theistic world view understand God's influence in different ways. These differences focus on how God works in creation, and a view of miracles.

These differences stem from the various characteristics of the modern world view. These characteristics are dualism, cause-and-effect, seeing change through the scientific method, and seeing creation as reliable.

The first difference, focusing on how God works in creation, believes that nature is "a rigidly determined mechanical order . . . a closed system of causal laws [that] excludes any belief in God's action in the world."[6] Christians who hold this view are likely to see God acting in their interpretation of events, not in the events themselves. Without God, we are likely to see the events in our lives as chaotic and meaningless. With God, we find hope because he enables us to give meaning and purpose to the events in our lives.

The second difference focuses on miracles. This difference affirms the influence of God on all creation. Yet it divides reality into physical and spiritual spheres, as Figure 2.3 illustrates. The natural elements of creation, which we can see, are separated from the supernatural elements of creation, which we cannot see. When God intervenes in nature, modern theists define the intervention, because it is out of the ordinary, as miraculous. It implies that God is not active in the natural operation of creation.

In organizing creation into physical and spiritual spheres, the modern theistic world view is dualistic. Dualism is a Greek idea that has had a profound influence on Western Christians. It has been a part of Western culture since Plato, a disciple of Socrates, wrote about it in about 350 B.C. Many early Christian theologians, particularly Augustine, were dualistic. Augustine called Plato "the most pure and bright in all of philosophy."[7] After his conversion to Christianity, Augustine, considered the fountainhead of Protestant and Catholic theology in the Western world, became an ascetic. He took a drastic turn from what he saw as the "evil of the material to the good of the spiritual soul."[8] René Descarte (1596-1650) finalized dualism by stating that the physical and spiritual realms of creation coexist, but do not interact.

Dualism continues to influence Christians in Western cultures. We continue to think of the unseen aspects of creation as spiritual and the seen as physical. These thoughts influence us to perceive the unseen spiritual realm as eternal and the seen physical realm as temporal. Yet the seen and the unseen aspects of creation are, in fact, created. Therefore, they cannot be eternal. Only God, the Creator, is eternal.

Dualism also influences how we perceive the composition of individual human beings. For example, ask Christians from Western cultures to explain the relationship between a person's physical body to the soul or spirit of the person. Most of them would use the "bird in the cage" analogy.[9] This analogy depicts an immortal spirit housed in a mortal body, as a bird is housed in a cage. At the death of the person—and possibly at other times—the spirit leaves the body. In doing so, the spirit experiences a freedom similar to the freedom a bird experiences upon its release from a cage.

Christians who separate evangelism from development have a dualistic world view. They use dualism to justify a "spiritual" ministry such as evangelism, instead of "physical" ministries in development. Such missionaries reason, "Why fix the cage when we really need to concentrate on the health of the bird?" Other missionaries agree that the cage needs fixing, but they designate this ministry as the second item on the agenda of Christian missions. The primary item is insuring the health of the birds.[10]

Modern Western theists see cause-and-effect within nature. In contrast to people with primal world views, however, they seek to find *how* something happened, instead of *why* it happened. They examine facts or events that they believe caused a particular change. For example, they understand illnesses in physical, not spiritual, terms. They believe that people get sick because they are infected with germs. Spirits, or people, did not send the germs to infect a person. Instead, germs cause illness because of conditions in the physical environment.

People who hold a Western theistic world view esteem the scientific method as the primary medium of change. They seek answers to inquiries that are methodological in nature. The answers to these inquiries have to be logically related to the cause-and-effect of the problem. Non-rational or transrational solutions have little credibility in Western world views. Western theists ask questions such as: Why are the elements in the environment arranged as they are? How can we manipulate or rearrange these elements to produce change?

The final characteristic of the Western theistic world view recognizes God's influence by acknowledging that his sovereign control makes the universe reliable. Because of this reliability, science is possible, and changes in the environment can be managed, manipulated and repeated.

The reliability of creation also leads modern people to accept risk. In contrast, people with primal world views are averse to risk. They do not see the environment as reliable, but as subject to the whims of the spirits.

The greatest contrast between the relational emphasis of primal world views and the cause-and-effect emphasis of modern theistic world views is how each accommodates spiritual intervention, or miracles. Since the integrity of the scientific method depends on non-intervention in an abnormal way by the Creator in creation, this world view has little room for miracles.

If Westerners experience miracles, they still believe that miracles have a methodological, cause-and-effect nature. This perception is probably not intentional, or even realized, but Westerners appear unable or unwilling to think otherwise. If modern theists experience a miraculous event, they are likely to attempt to replicate the condition in which the event occurred to reproduce the miracle.

In contrast to the Western world view, miracles are normal for the primal world view. In some cultures, the idea that God intervenes in nature is so commonplace that the people probably do not have a word for this intervention. A word for *miracle* is superfluous; belief in the existence of God assumes he intervenes in nature. It is granted along with his existence.

Implications of these world views on missions

As the stories in chapter one showed, power as the central organizing theme of primal world views prevents people who hold these world views from focusing on the ultimate meanings and purposes of life. Instead, it reduces faith to utilitarian values that put people in an either-or quandary. The relationships the people have with the spirits are either powerful enough, or not powerful enough, to influence the spirits to change the present circumstances of life. If people with primal world views want their circumstances to change, they must either develop stronger relationships with the spiritual powers or reconcile themselves to accept circumstances that are beyond the control or interest of the spiritual realm.

If we applied the assumptions of primal world views to Christianity, the end result would communicate that God has limited sovereignty. This results from his limited power over or interest in creation, or because he is competing with adversaries for control of a particular situation or for the entire creation.

In both situations, Christians are in the position of reconciling themselves to a limited God, or appeasing God to persuade him to express his power in particular instances. This world view reduces worship to a variety of rituals for building a relationship with God so we can influence his will or power to get particular results. Either situation prevents Christians from realizing the regenerative nature of God's covenantal relationship with creation.

The modern theistic world view solves the problem of God expressing or not expressing his power or interest in particular situations by separating physical enterprises from spiritual enterprises. People with this world view do not expect God to intervene in nature. If he does, they appreciate his intervention—but usually verify it with science. If he does not intervene, the basic assumptions of the world view are not challenged.

This solution creates more problems than it solves. It results in a dichotomy that separates the physical from the spiritual, the natural from the supernatural, the sacred from the secular, the facts from values, and the public from the private (see Figure 2.5 below).

Most of us, if we have any sense of integration, have trouble with this classification. In most situations, facts cannot be used apart from values and the public and personal spheres blend and overlap. The distinction between sacred and secular is artificial, and the natural-supernatural distinction does not adequately explain how God works in creation. God's redemptive work is not either natural or supernatural, it is both natural

Figure 2.5   The dichotomy caused by the modern world view

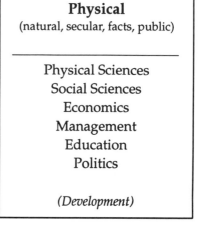

Spiritual	**Physical**
(supernatural, sacred, values, private)	(natural, secular, facts, public)
Theology	Physical Sciences
Religion	Social Sciences
Ethics	Economics
	Management
	Education
	Politics
(Evangelism)	*(Development)*

and supernatural. This both-and understanding of God's redemptive work erases the dichotomy.

If we look at particular pursuits that Christian ministry engages in, we also would find the dichotomy inadequate. Economics—classified as *the worldly philosophy*,[11] a label given to the study by its founders—falls on the physical side of the dichotomy. Yet the distribution of resources cannot be free of ethics or values. Addressing the creation and distribution of resources in a culture is unavoidably spiritual. *Shalom* cannot be realized without the just distribution of resources.

Ecology is undoubtedly a physical science, but we cannot address it apart from theological, religious or ethical issues. The choice to invest time or money in ecological efforts has spiritual implications. It challenges us to ask whether we are investing in them because they are fashionable or because we have a high view of creation. We are making a spiritual statement either way. We either want our faith to be fashionable or we want to honor God by caring for his handiwork.

Modern theists think of medicine as a physical pursuit because it focuses on the body, not the spirit. Yet it has spiritual implications, particularly if people think of healing as a supernatural act. But most medical professionals and patients do not want to see their treatment as either-or. It is both physical and spiritual; it transcends the dichotomy we tend to put it in. Medicine is effective not only because of its ability to restore physical bodies to health. It is effective also because the Creator of these bodies enables them to be restored to health.

Social sciences such as sociology, political science, and education are classified as physical. Christians attempt to sanctify or spiritualize them by giving them a Christian adjective: Christian economics or Christian psychology. This implies that the values of Christian social sciences differ from the values of non-Christian social sciences.

But flavoring social sciences with Christian values does not change the nature of the subjects. Whether we flavor the subjects with Christian or other values, they cannot be value-free. Therefore, we cannot isolate or restrict their influence on our lives. Values cannot be restricted to the private, sacred area of life, and facts cannot be the only determining factors in the public and secular spheres. Life simply cannot be carved up so neatly.

The physical-spiritual dichotomy has a profound impact on how we perceive the missiological task of the church.

For example, development and evangelism come on opposite sides of the natural-supernatural dichotomy of the modern theistic world view. So modern theists frequently pit one against the other. Development meets physical needs, possibly at the expense of meeting spiritual ones. Evangelism brings eternal hope to people at the expense of living their temporal lives in despair.

According to the modern theistic world view, people who accept Christ because of development projects are vulnerable to being seen as *rice Christians*. They profess faith in Christ because their physical needs are being met. If you asked the people who come to Christ because of development projects why they became Christians, in their ignorance of the physical-spiritual dichotomy they might say "because the missionaries have given us rice."

This response is an anathema. The converts are enjoying physical blessings apart from a spiritual commitment to the Blesser. Evangelism, an effort to get people on the spiritual side of the dichotomy, is defeated. In this scenario, development has little redemptive value. It leads people who were once ripe for spiritual nourishment to corruption, or even secularization, by the materialism that development fostered. Development did not bring people closer to the kingdom of God. Instead, it left them blissfully enjoying the physical fruits of a developed, modernized society.

Let us examine another answer to the question, "Why did you become a Christian?" A person appealing to the natural-supernatural dichotomy may say, "Christianity enabled me to develop an ethical code to govern my behavior." This response seems more acceptable than the response to receiving rice. Ethics, reflecting some spiritual values, fall on the spiritual side of the dichotomy.

Yet do ethics bear witness to God's empowerment more effectively than food does? The behavior of the Pharisees we read about in the Gospels seems to show that ethics can become another blessing separated from the Blesser. The ethics of the Pharisees were impeccable, but the New Testament shows that ethics did not lead the Pharisees to a healthy relationship with God. If we erased the physical-spiritual dichotomy from Western culture, we would probably not believe that *ethics Christians* are more pleasing to God than *rice Christians*.

A holistic world view mediates the clash

If we examine the Bible to understand how it relates to the primal or modern world views, we will find elements of both world views in it. In the Bible, as in primal world views, relationships between God and the prophets cause miracles to happen, affirming God's intervention in nature. Seas part, bushes burn without being consumed, people follow clouds to discern God's guidance, and God even speaks through Balaam's donkey.

We also can interpret the Bible to affirm the understanding that health and illness have relational causes in the spiritual sense. On a general level, through Adam's fall—which fractured his relationship with God—sin and death entered the world. Consequently, people live under the curse of sin, and suffer illnesses and death as consequences of sin.

On a particular level, we also can attribute illnesses and death to a relationship with God. Theologians understand that Saul's illness came from an "evil spirit from the Lord" (1 Sam. 19:9). Similarly, the disciples of Jesus initially believed a blind man suffered from the effects of his sin or the sins of his parents. Also, Ananias and Sapphira died of God's curse when they lied to the Holy Spirit about withholding from the community some of the money from the sale of their land (Acts 5:1-5).

From the perspective of a Western world view, you can show biblical support for a more moderate view of God's extraordinary intervention in creation. According to this world view, the general effects of Adam's curse are real, but the particular effects of the curse are more indirect. People are not victims of divine whim, but they suffer from the consequences of their behavior. Those who hold this view might say that Ananias and Sapphira suffered from their inability to live peacefully in their community.

People with a modern, theistic world view think the Hebrews believed that Saul had an evil spirit from God because they had no other way of categorizing his insanity. Those who hold this view also believe Jesus corrected the apostles when they asked if the man was blind because of his sin or the sins of his parents. Jesus said: "Neither this man nor his parents sinned, but this happened so the work of God might be displayed in this life" (John 9:3). Apparently, the man was blind so God could be glorified.

The question for the Western theistic world view is whether the healings and other miracles of Jesus are normal or exceptional. Some biblical teachings and narratives indicate that miracles are exceptional. For example, God chose not to remove the thorn in Paul's flesh, and Paul prescribed wine, a physical cure, for Timothy's stomach ailment. Luke, the great physician, marvelled at the miracles of Jesus and the apostles. If these incidents were normal, Luke might not have paid so much attention to them.

Discussing the biblical preference for a primal or Western world view is not as useful as finding a third alternative. Since we seldom find truth in synthesis, we do not prefer a third alternative that synthesizes the two common world views. Instead, we want a world view that organizes reality around the covenant that God has made with creation. That world view, like the covenant, is organized around *shalom*.

Figure 2.6 (see page 30) illustrates a biblical, holistic world view. It is distinct from the Western world view because it does not organize the

Figure 2.6[12]   Hebraic-Holistic world view

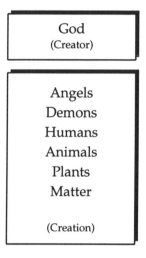

universe around the seen or unseen, physical or spiritual, sacred or secular. Also, unlike the primal world view, God is not a part of creation. Instead, this world view organizes the universe to recognize the distinction between God and creation. The created elements, whether seen or unseen, are mortal and fallen. They exist apart from the uncreated Creator.[13]

The basis for this world view is a belief that God is working redemptively through the entire creation. It shows that God and his people are working toward restoring the elements of creation to fulfill the purposes for which they were created. While this world view is evident throughout the entire canon, Colossians 1:15-20 depicts it especially well. In this passage, Paul affirms that "all things were created: things in heaven and on earth, visible and invisible" (Col. 1:16), and "through him [Jesus] to reconcile to himself all things, whether things on earth or things in heaven, by making peace through his blood, shed on the cross" (Col. 1:20).

If we read Colossians 1:15-20 from the assumptions of a primal world view, the passage would make little sense. The primal world view, which sees the universe as a seamless garment, does not lend itself to appreciating the impact of the Creator reconciling creation to himself. People with a primal world view perceive the Creator, knowingly or unknowingly, as part of creation.

The passage has greater implications for the Western theistic world view. We who hold this world view are prone to thinking that the visible and invisible elements of creation have different natures. We believe that the visible elements of creation have physical natures, and creation's invisible elements have spiritual natures. Placing the unseen elements of creation in the spiritual dimension of reality leads us to believe, perhaps unconsciously, that the unseen elements of creation are somehow uncreated, or eternal. This belief gives the unseen elements of creation a nature that is different from the nature of the seen, or physical, elements of creation.

The Western theistic world view also implies that the unseen elements of creation, being spiritual, are of the same nature as the Creator. It fails to acknowledge the explicit distinction the Bible makes between the nature of creation and that of the Creator. Instead, it forms a dichotomy between the physical and spiritual dimensions of creation, putting the Creator in the same category as the unseen elements of creation.

The holistic world view erases the dichotomy in creation that the dualistic Western world view produces. It does this by affirming that God sustains and redeems the seen and the unseen elements of creation. It does not view the visible elements of creation as physical or the unseen elements of creation as spiritual. Instead, it acknowledges that all created elements, whether they are seen or unseen, solid, liquid or gaseous, material or immaterial, will be reconciled to the Creator.

Biblical holism regards many human activities as part of God's reconciling work in creation. It does not distinguish any discipline or pursuit as physical or spiritual, but values all activities for their contribution to redeeming a fallen creation. Economics, medicine and agriculture, for example, are valued for the contributions they make to ministries that participate in God's redemptive work in creation.

Holism also enables us to perceive God's role in creation as normal, not miraculous. Holism does not set aside events that appear to witness to God's intervention in nature, the physical realm of creation. Instead, it acknowledges that God works in creation in general and particular ways. Generally, he works through the laws of nature that he endowed in creation. He also works in particular situations by intervening in these laws. In both situations, God works to reconcile creation to himself.

Contrasting the dualistic and holistic world views

Since dualism is so pervasive in Western culture and in the missions community, some contrasts between the assumptions of dualism and holism are worth noting.

In contrast to dualism, holism does not affirm the bird in the cage analogy. It does not see the human body as having immortal and mortal aspects that separate after death. Instead, it affirms the Hebraic belief that the spiritual dimension of creation, particularly the spiritual dimension of the human being, is not, by nature, immortal. The Hebrews never separated the body and soul, and the spiritual could not outlive the physical.

In Hebrew thought the body, animated by the soul, constituted the human being. When Stephen told the Sanhedrin that 75 souls went to Egypt, he did not think the souls had an existence apart from the body. He was telling the Sanhedrin that 75 animated bodies went to Egypt (Acts 7:14, RSV). Westerners continue to use the word "soul" in this way. When we say, "There wasn't a soul in the house," we are not saying bodies were present without souls. Instead, we are emphasizing that no one was in the house.

The second assumption the Hebrews made about the soul was that it was mortal. In contrast to the Greeks, the Hebrews did not think their souls could outlive their bodies. When the body died, the soul ceased to exist. Jesus seemed to affirm this point. During his agony at Gethsemane he said to his disciples, "My soul is overwhelmed with sorrow to the point of death" (Matt. 26:38).

This second assumption is vital to understanding the place of death and resurrection in the holistic world view of the Hebrews. In contrast to the Greeks, the Hebrews did not think that death released the bird from the cage, showing a transition from mortal life to eternal life. Instead, the Hebrews understood that death caused a person's existence to cease. They believed that the resurrection overcame death by raising the deceased person to new life. In Hebrew thought a person did not go from life to life, but went from life to death to a new, resurrected life.

The deaths of Socrates and Jesus illustrate the difference between Greek dualistic thought and the holistic thought of the Hebrews.

Phaedo, a disciple of Socrates, recorded the discourse that Socrates delivered to his disciples on the day he died. In his discourse, Socrates serenely spoke of philosophical issues as he approached his death. Socrates did not fear death, but looked forward to releasing the bird from the cage. The disciples who heard his message had more grief over his death than he did. Socrates saw his death as a transition from an incarnated soul to a disembodied one.

The writers of the Gospels did not portray the death of Jesus so serenely. Unlike Socrates, Jesus did not welcome death as a transition that liberated his soul from his body; Jesus anguished over his death. He anticipated that the resurrection would eventually overcome death, but he still saw death overcoming life. In contrast to Socrates, who saw death as the passage to eternal life, Jesus saw death as death, with the resurrection bringing new life.

Do we follow the village shaman, Socrates or Jesus?

We face modeling our ministries after the village shaman, Socrates or Jesus in the contrasts between creating Christian ministry after primal, dualistic or holistic world views. In a Socratic sense, we can see the pain and suffering that people experience in this life as incidental to their spiritual welfare. Or, like the village shaman, we could see ourselves as brokers of God's power as it is displayed in our efforts to bring healing to a fractured world. From the holistic world view, however, we see ourselves participating in the redemptive work of Christ.

We are not brokers of God's power or bearers of a message that separates the physical and spiritual dimensions of God's creation. Instead, we see ourselves called by God to work redemptively in the entire creation. The village shaman, in contrast, is not seeking redemption in creation. His concern is with appeasing the elements of the spiritual realm. He appeases the spirits to manipulate the elements of creation to his advantage. He sees creation as the domain of the spirits, instead of believing that he, himself, has dominion over it.

Socrates, like the village shaman, also cared little about the physical aspects of his humanity or the physical elements of creation. Unlike later Greek philosophers, he did not see creation as necessarily evil. Instead, he saw it as the arena of the gods who cared only about their self-interest. He did not attempt to appease the gods for particular outcomes; he saw such attempts as foolishness. Instead, he perceived a world that could be organized around human thought and reason.

Socrates said, "The unexamined life is not worth living." He dedicated his life to reason and introspection as he examined and perfected the immortal soul that he believed his mortal body contained. If he had lived during the time of Jesus' ministry, Socrates would have been confused as to why Jesus bothered to heal the sick, feed the hungry and raise the dead. In his dualistic view, the physical nature of humanity did not contribute to the ultimate purpose of life, but frustrated it.

Jesus, unlike Socrates or the village shaman, saw the entire creation participating in the redemptive work of God. He believed creation was good because God, its Creator, was good. He did not see that evil—the cause of creation's fallen nature—and the goodness of God were diametrically opposed. Instead, he saw evil within the context of God's redemptive work.

Paul seems to have exercised this view of evil when he instructed the Corinthians to "hand this man over to Satan, so that the sinful nature may be destroyed and his spirit saved on the day of the Lord" (1 Cor. 5:5). Similarly, he seems to tell Timothy that he handed Hymenaeus and Alexander "over to Satan to be taught not to blaspheme" (1 Tim. 1:20).

From the perspective of Socrates, or a form of Greek dualism imposed on Christianity, Paul is like a general who turns his treasonous troops over to the enemy. This way, the traitors will become more useful to the loyal troops. In this world view, Paul's integrity falls apart.

In contrast to a dualistic world view, a holistic world view enables us to salvage Paul's integrity. Holism can hold good and evil together because it recognizes the relationship of the Creator to creation. In holism, creation is one reality, both spiritual and physical, good and bad. It includes "things in heaven and on earth, visible and invisible, whether thrones or powers or rulers or authorities" (Col. 1:16). In the holistic world view, evil and Satan (the personification of evil) are subject to God, who ultimately determines what Satan is permitted to do. Like Satan's role in the Book of Job, when God said to Satan, "Very well, then, everything [Job] has is in your hands, but on the man himself do not lay a finger" (Job 1:12), holism sees Satan in the role of the accuser, tempter, deceiver and destroyer. Yet his role in creation and his work are not beyond the redemptive power of God.

Holism affirms Walter Wink's view, who wrote, "We must never attempt to straitjacket Satan in rigid doctrinal categories. Satan is not a fixed, unnuanced figure."[14] Neither does a holistic Christian world view reject the radicalness of evil. Instead, holism sees the redemptive power of God reconciling the interdependent elements of creation to himself.

Integrating holism and Christian missions

Christian development agencies that worked in a particular East African culture vividly portrayed the need to integrate a holistic Christian world view with Christian missions.

Animistic farmers inhabited the region. Each year before the planting season, they gathered on their fields to perform a ceremony that they believed appeased the spirits that controlled the land. In the ceremony, hundreds of men gathered at each end of the field, then rushed toward the middle of the field to beat each other with freshly cut tree branches. The shedding of blood was an offering to the spirits that the farmers believed made the land productive.

Bodily injuries were countless. Noses were broken, eyes were injured, and teeth fell out. Still, the farmers thought of the pain and suffering as small investments in comparison to the abundant harvests that the blood brought. If people considered the pain and suffering unreasonable, they should consider the effects of starvation, the result of land that gives no crops because it has no blood.

Christian and non-Christian Western development agencies came to the community to implement agricultural programs. Agronomists analyzed soils, recommended fertilizers, and brought in drought-resistant seeds. With varying degrees of success, the agronomists introduced new crops, and the community realized increased yields in other crops.

Yet, ironically, the community and the Christian development practitioners became ambivalent toward the programs for the same reason. Both groups saw spirituality as a problem, but the problem stemmed from different world views, not different expressions of spirituality.

The people who lived in the village had a pragmatic view of spirituality. They saw that their livelihood depended on their making peace with the spirits that delivered abundant agricultural harvests. If crops failed, the community had to understand why the spirits were angry. If crops succeeded, the community attributed success to the moods of the spirits.

The villagers were averse to risk. They did not want to jeopardize their relationships with the spirits by putting their faith in the chemicals of the agronomists. Can the chemicals produce rain? they wondered. Can chemicals work if rain does not come? Who is the spirit behind the chemicals? Is the spirit of the chemicals more powerful than the local spirits?

In contrast to the villagers, the holistic development practitioners thought the community had a misguided spirituality. The development practitioners did not believe that the spirits, or any spiritual realm, had a tangible influence on agriculture. The spirits did not fit into the agriculture methods that grew out of the Western world view. The Christian development practitioners who held this world view deliberately separated their spiritual calling from their development work. The community, in contrast, could not see the benefit of a religion that did not produce tangible results.

There was a holistic solution to the dilemma these groups faced. The Christian development practitioners could have applied the communion sacrament, the central rite of Christianity, to their agricultural context. Christianity affirms the sacrifice of Christ as the final sacrifice for the sins of humankind. As the ultimate sacrifice, it reconciles people and creation to God.

If they had celebrated communion in the church building, or preferably in the fields at the beginning of planting season, the community could have made the connection between Christ's sacrifice and the spiritual dimension of agriculture. Both the development practitioners and the villagers could then see that God enables them to embrace a different world view. The villagers would find release from their bondage to the spirits, and the missionaries could integrate their work and their message. Each would see *shalom* as the unifying agent that symbolizes the redemptive work of God, through Christ, in creation.

Answering the questions people are asking

I encountered a similar situation in Ghana. Christianity has become part of the fabric of Ghanaian culture, but it has not taken significant root in it. Christianity is more of a veneer over many traditional Ghanaian beliefs. In the *National Church Survey*, the Ghana Evangelism Committee noted that "over 60 percent of all Ghanaians and 70-80 percent of those in Southern Ghana" claim to be Christians.[15] Yet the "national average church attendance is 11 percent."[16]

There is a widespread belief that a lack of discipleship causes the disparity between the number of apparent conversions and church attendance. We say that the likely solution to this problem is emphasizing personal evangelism and discipleship. While these disciplines are valuable, we invariably define them according to a Western world view. This perspective causes us to miss the issues that make Christianity relevant in Ghana and other primal cultures. For example, the discipleship materials were developed in Europe and North America. These materials prevent the gospel from answering the questions the people are asking. They also decontextualize worship and make church attendance irrelevant.

The missionaries who brought Christianity to Ghana—and to many other African cultures—had a strategy of "mission by extension."[17] They assumed that the issues that emerged from developing a Christian spirituality in a Western culture also could extend to primal cultures. For example, the missionaries were concerned with personal salvation, the forgiveness of sin and living sanctified lives. They taught the Ghanaians such truths as "all have sinned and fall short of the glory of God" (Rom. 3:23), and "the wages of sin is death, but the gift of God is eternal life in Christ Jesus our Lord" (Rom. 6:23).

While these truths are important, they did not position the missionaries to speak to the situations of the villagers. The missionaries communicated the spirituality of Christianity in a more abstract manner. Their message reflected a world view in which the seen and unseen worlds were less likely to interact with each other.

The questions the people in the village asked did not assume an abstract spirituality. They believed the unseen world governed changes in the seen world.

The villagers believed the power of any spirituality had to manifest itself tangibly in the physical world. Not that sin, salvation and sanctification did not matter to them, but they developed a spiritual framework that emerged from their need for such things as food, water, health, and fertility. Their concern with physical issues was not at the expense of spiritual issues. Instead, they saw physical issues as intensely spiritual.

Some basic world view assumptions separated the missionaries and the villagers. The holistic, biblical world view, in addressing salvation as an ingredient of *shalom*, bridges the gap between the world views of the missionaries and the villagers. Christ's redemptive work applies to all of creation. By placing the salvation message within this context, the holistic, biblical world view communicates this message in a way that answers the questions the people are asking. It does not create a dichotomy between meeting the physical and spiritual needs of the people. Instead, it recognizes that redemption addresses the seen and the unseen elements of creation, making development work intrinsically evangelistic and relevant in primal cultures.

Interpreting development work within a spiritual framework

Let's use a well-drilling project to illustrate how the redemptive work of Christ in creation makes development work intrinsically evangelistic. The point of the following story is to show how the villagers—many of whom were Christians—interpreted the meaning of the wells within a spiritual framework. Even so, they could not hold their spiritual interpretation of the wells and their Christian faith together.

The villagers' world view assumed a spiritual interpretation of the wells, but they did not see Christianity providing a way for them to make that interpretation. Accordingly, they interpreted the spiritual meaning of the wells in the context of their traditional religion. The wells—and the accompanying community development projects—reinforced the two separate realities the villagers had to contend with. In the words of Tite Tiénou, the people in the village experienced "the tremendous burden of having to bear at least two cultural loads: the modern or so-called Western, and the traditional . . . the center can hold no longer . . ."[18] A holistic, biblical world view can transform the traditional world view, enabling the people to hold the spiritual interpretation of the wells with the message of personal salvation.

The primary assumption of the indigenous world view is that the natural water sources have spiritual power. "Almost all West African communities believe that there are deities inhabiting the waters," wrote Kofi Asare Opoku.[19] Rivers, streams or water holes are the spiritual centers of Ghanaian villages.

The people also affirm the existence of a god who resides in heaven. Ghanaian Christians and non-Christians assert that this god is the same deity that the Christians worship. But the "river is also god."[20] God exists in the river, as the river, and apart from the river. Also, the river is not the water; the river gives water, but it exists apart from the water.

People in the villages invariably affirm the divine power of the river. Yet there is some ambivalence about the nature of the river's power. Non-Christians do not assign a value to the power of the river. It is neither good nor bad, but is both good and bad. It has the power to give water, the substance of life, and the power to take life: people drown in it.

The Christians in the village perceived the power of the river more ambivalently. Some of them believed the river had no power; most were willing to admit that the river had power. Still, they were ambivalent about the nature of the power and its source. Some believed the river had power because it was satanic or evil. Others believed the river had power because God gave it power.

Because the river had power, there were regulations for drawing water from it. These regulations prohibited people from getting water on the day of the week that the river was created, or born. Menstruating women were forbidden from getting water, and people could not use dirty or black pots to draw water from the river. People were also forbidden from catching fish, frogs or crabs from their section of the river (yet they could harvest fish, frogs and crabs from another section of the river). Both Christians and non-Christians observed these regulations: some out of spiritual obligation and others because of social cohesion.

When a team from a Christian development agency entered the village to discuss preparations for well-drilling, the villagers faced a problem. They believed the river would be offended—and would possibly withhold water—if they allowed well-drilling without its permission. The villagers also knew that the well-drilling team did not affirm the power of the river. The people on the drilling team prayed, but they did not address their prayers to the river. The villagers did not believe that prayers from people who did not affirm the river's power could appease the river.

The village elders solved the dilemma by making sacrifices of animals or palm wine to seek permission for well-drilling from the river. The people believed that the river had accepted their sacrifices if the drilling team struck water. In most situations, the villagers believed the river benevolently accepted their sacrifices by giving water to the boreholes.

In other situations, the river was not as benevolent. The boreholes were dry. After the drilling team failed to strike water in one village, the village elders went to the river to make a sacrifice. The next borehole was wet. The people concluded that the river gave permission for the second borehole in response to their sacrifice.

I was part of a group that visited several of the villages that now have wells. When we asked the villagers what they thought about the wells, they became enthusiastic about how the wells had improved the quality of their lives. They and their children were healthier; they saw improvements in their personal hygiene and nutrition, and the number of water-borne diseases had dropped. An added pleasure was that, unlike the river, there were no regulations about drawing water from the wells. The women could go to the wells any day of the week and any time of the month. They also could carry well water in any type of pot. Invariably, the people believed the wells were the best improvement made to their communities.

Then we asked the villagers why the wells had been drilled. We expected the answers to reflect the spiritual values of the well-drilling team—answers such as, "Christians are drilling wells in our villages because God loves us." However, the question did not mean much to the villagers. The connection between the wells and the love of the God proclaimed by the drilling team did not speak to the people. They agreed with the statement, but it did not address their view of reality.

We changed the question to inquire how the people understood the relationship between the wells and the rivers. This question was meaningful; the people invariably responded that the water in the wells was the gift of the river. Many village elders made annual sacrifices to the river so the river would continue to give water to the wells.

While the Christians in the villages were more ambivalent about the river's power, they also believed the water in the wells was a gift from the river. In one village, the Christians agreed that they should not participate in the sacrifices the community elders made to the river. Still, it pleased them that the elders made the sacrifices because they did not want the river to use its power to withhold water from the wells.

As Christians with a Western world view, we did not separate the water from the wells. Yet the people in the villages thought the wells were incidental to the water. They knew the Christians from an agency in the capital city drilled wells for the glory of God, but this did not impress them. The wells were only as good as the water in them; they were meaningless if the river did not provide water for them. Further, the wells did not bear witness to the Good News of Jesus Christ. Instead, they gave the villagers an opportunity to affirm the benevolent power of the river.

Wells, rivers and God's redemptive work in creation

We can use this story to illustrate how development has a detrimental effect on evangelism, but it also shows how a good project needs a good interpretation. If we want the people to understand that the wells bring Good News to their villages, we must start with the river. We must show how the river is part of a fallen creation, and how creation has a Savior who calls us to participate in his work of redeeming it. The wells, then, become a symbol of God's redemptive work in creation. They are an answer to the pragmatic problem of getting clean water in a fallen creation. They also provide an opportunity to communicate the need for personal salvation. Finally, they are a reminder that God calls people to practice justice in society.

While the indigenous people believe the river has divine power, this belief is not far from the Christian idea that the river, as part of creation, reflects the power of God. At one time the river gave pure water that sustained the life God breathed into all human beings. Yet the river, because of the Fall, became polluted; the water was no longer fit to drink. The ability of the water to sustain life deteriorated to the point where drinking the water caused people to get sick. If people drink the river water now, they can get a variety of diseases and will possibly die.

Yet sickness and death are not the end of the story. God's answer to the fallen creation was to redeem it to enable it to support life, to fulfill his purposes for it. He sent his Son, the Savior, who died on the cross and was resurrected, to redeem all creation. Through the crucifixion of Jesus Christ, the progressive redemption of creation occurs in several ways.

Wells are one expression of a progressively redeemed creation. They are a result of God inspiring people to gain the knowledge to understand how the effects of the Fall can be reversed. God enables us to drill wells that give clean water in response to a river that gives dirty water. God inspires us to seek life in a creation that is slanted toward death.

The wells provide water that improves every area of our lives. It enables people to be cleaner and healthier; it improves medical care and agricultural harvest; it eases the burden of daily chores and improves social relationships. These factors are part of God's plan for the redemption of creation. While the river represents a fallen creation, the wells bear witness to God's love for creation, and his willingness to redeem it.

The wells also serve as redemptive analogies to communicate the presence of sin in our lives and the need for salvation and sanctification. But the wells are more than analogies. They bear witness, in a culturally relevant manner, that God's redemptive work is not only concerned with redeeming the physical world—it also extends to redeeming the human condition.

Like the river, people are also affected by the Fall. We do not live as God intended for us to live, but we live according to our fallen natures. While the Fall caused the river to yield water that causes sickness and death, our behavior also causes sickness, social disharmony and, eventually, death. We no longer live to fulfill the purposes for which God created us. Our sin leads to death, but the redemptive work of God through Jesus Christ gives us life.

Our current state of sinfulness is not the end of the story. The redemptive work of Christ frees us from sin. It enables us to live lives that overcome the effects of sin—sin from our personal and social conditions—and to participate in God's desire to resurrect us into eternal life after death.

Wells also facilitate redemption at the structural level. People created structures in society as the mechanisms for providing order. In chapter nine we will deal more extensively with this issue. It is sufficient to say here that all structures are fallen, and they affect cultural values such as the division of labor, the use of time, and the stewardship of natural resources. They too are elements of creation that participate in the redemptive work of Christ.

Wells affect the social order in a community to the extent that they speak to the structures in a community. In the Ghanaian villages, the wells influence the concept of a sabbath, the division of labor, and the stewardship of natural resources. Before the installation of the wells, the regulations concerning the river were the structures that provided order. The river regulations required a day of rest for women who carried containers of water that weigh as much as 70 pounds. There were regulations providing a few days of rest for women when they were menstruating. River regulations also insured the use of clean water containers, and set some directives about harvesting fish from the river.

In contrast, there were no regulations concerning the wells. The people celebrated their freedom from the river's regulations, but they may not have been better off. Yes, the women could get water any day of the week or month—resulting in added work for them. The villagers could now get away with using dirty containers, and the well had little influence over their use of natural resources.

To suggest the transfer of the river regulations to the wells would insult our sense of Christian liberty by enslaving the people to laws. Yet we can transform the river regulations to reflect the redeemed structures that insure a justly ordered environment and displays our liberty in Christ.

For example, our Christian liberty enables us to enjoy a day of rest. It gives us a sense of justice that enables us to divide labor fairly. Our Christian liberty also enables us to be effective stewards of creation. We do not carry water in dirty pots because we know that creation is full of germs that will contaminate the water. We do not indiscriminately harvest fish and other natural resources, because they are part of an ordered creation. We can harvest them to a point, but only if they can be replenished.

Communicating God's redemptive work through symbols

The final issue is how we can effectively communicate this some-what abstract reasoning to the people in the villages. The best way to do so is through symbols. Traditionally, the people sacrificed animals and poured out libations of palm wine to get the river's permission for the wells. The Christians in Ghana, as elsewhere, have the elements of the eucharist, a dynamic equivalent to the traditional libations. The libations symbolize the temporal sacrifice of the traditional religion. The communion elements symbolize the eternal sacrifice of Christ. The elements of communion serve as concrete symbols for communicating and celebrating God's redemptive work in creation. They symbolize the final sacrifice Christ made for the redemption of all elements in creation.

If over 80 percent of Ghanaian Christians are not attending churches,[21] then discipleship programs are essential, but they must be based on the questions the people are asking. The people care about forgiveness, sanctification and salvation, but these issues express themselves differently in that culture. Discipleship programs must address reality as the traditional world view depicts it. They must then work toward transforming that perception and enabling the people to see how their perception of reality fits into a holistic, biblical world view.

Can wells communicate that the redemptive work of Christ includes personal salvation, social justice and environmental responsibility? They can if we interpret them effectively. The issue is not providing a spiritual interpretation of development where there is none. Instead, it is realizing that people in many cultures interpret development according to their traditional world views unless they have a reason not to make such an interpretation.

Biblical holism provides a way for people to interpret their personal salvation in the context of the redemption of all creation. God did not limit redemption to one dimension of creation. Biblical holism transforms our world views, enabling us to understand that God brings peace to every aspect of creation through the redemptive work of Christ.

NOTES

1. Benezet Buju, *African Theology in its Social Context* (Maryknoll: Orbis Books, 1992), p. 31.

2. These diagrams are based on illustrations found in *Phenomenology and Institutions of Folk Religions*, Paul G. Hiebert (Pasadena: Fuller Theological Seminary, 1990), pp. 16 and 22.

3. Buju, p. 20.

4. Paul H. Hiebert, "The Flaw of the Excluded Middle," *Missiology: An International Review*, Vol. 10:1 (January 1982): 35-47.

5. David Burnett, *Unearthly Powers: A Christian Perspective on Primal and Folk Religions* (Eastbourne: MARC/Monarch Publications, Ltd., 1988), p. 8.

6. Ian G. Barbour, *Science and Secularity: The Ethics of Technology* (New York: Harper and Row, 1970), p. 39.

7. Diogenes Allen, *Philosophy for Understanding Theology* (Atlanta: John Knox Press, 1985), p. 81.

8. David G. Myers, *The Human Puzzle: Psychological Research and Christian Belief* (New York: Harper and Row, 1978), p. 81.

9. This assumption is based on a survey cited on p. 73 of *The Human Puzzle* by David G. Myers (see Note 8 above). While this survey is dated, it is still valid because attitudes toward religious beliefs, as evidenced by the research of George Gallup, change slowly.

10. Articles such as those by Jim Yost and Ralph C. Owens support this view of Christian missions. In *Why the World Waits: Exposing the Reality of Modern Missions*, K. P. Yohannan suggests "missions have somehow been deliberately sabotaged by a 'satanic plot'" (p. 101).

11. Taken from the title of the book by Robert L. Heilbroner, *The Worldly Philosophers* (New York: Simon and Schuster, 1986).

12. From an illustration in Hiebert, 1990, p. 22. Demons in the holistic world view can be defined as non-material, fallen entities or as metaphors to describe fallen structures in society. Chapter nine will address this point in more detail.

13. This distinction is not to imply that God is withdrawn from creation, but it is to acknowledge that the uncreated nature of God distinguishes him from the created nature of spiritual and physical beings. This distinction between the separate existences of God and creation is vitally important to understanding a biblical view of holism. It highlights the difference between the uncreated nature of God and the created nature of the universe. If the distinction was not made, a Christian form of pantheism would result. Philip M. Steyne makes this point in *Gods of Power: A Study of the Beliefs and Practices of Animists* (Houston: Touch Publications, 1990), p. 59. He states: "Holism is foundational to animism and leads logically to pantheism." While this statement is undoubtedly true for non-biblical views of holism, it does not reflect the nature of biblical holism.

14. Walter Wink, *Unmasking the Powers: The Invisible Forces that Determine Human Existence* (Philadelphia: Fortress Press, 1986), p. 33.

15. Ghana Evangelism Committee (GEC), *National Church Survey: Facing the Unfinished Task of the Church in Ghana* (Accra, Ghana: GEC, 1989), p. 5.

16. Ibid.

17. The phrase "mission by extension" emerged in a seminar in Accra, Ghana, led by Merrill Ewert.

18. Tite Tiénou, *The Theological Task of the Church in Africa* (Achimota, Ghana: Africa Christian Press, 1990), p.22.

19. Kofi Asare Opoku, *West African Traditional Religion* (Accra, Ghana: FEP International, 1978), p. 60.

20. Agnes Phillips, "When Tradition Resists Development," *People's Daily Graphic*, Accra, Ghana (December 14, 1992): 5.

21. This figure is based on 11 percent of the people attending church while over 60 percent have made a commitment to Christ: (60-11)/60 = 82 percent.

THREE

Contextualization:
Communicating good news

Paul then stood up
in the meeting of the Areopagus and said:
"Men of Athens!
I see that in every way you are very religious.
For as I walked around
and observed your objects of worship,
I even found an altar with the inscription:
TO AN UNKNOWN GOD.
Now what you worship as something unknown
I am going to proclaim to you."
Acts 17:22-23

At that, Paul left the Council.
A few men became followers of Paul and believed. . . .
Acts 17:33-34a

CONTEXTUALIZATION IS AN EFFORT to understand the frames of reference and world views that people have developed to make sense out of their environment.

The apostle Paul contextualized his message when he visited Athens. When meeting the Athenians, he referred to their altar that had an inscription TO AN UNKNOWN GOD. Apparently the Athenians wanted to have inscriptions to every known deity, but did not have the confidence that they knew every deity. They attempted to solve their dilemma by making an inscription to the god who possibly existed, but whom they did not know.

Paul saw this inscription as an indicator of what the Athenians would see as good news: making the unknown god known. After Paul introduced the unknown God to the Athenians, some of them responded to his message by coming to faith in the God that Paul proclaimed. Others wanted to learn more about that God.

When Christians from the West encounter people of other cultures, both Christians and non-Christians, contextual issues invariably surface. The central question asks how the holistic nature of the gospel can be relevant to particular cultural contexts without filtering it through Western or primal world views. To this end, contextualization attempts to tell the truth of the gospel by making it culturally relevant without having it become culturally relative.

The following stories illustrate some problems that can occur without contextualization.

The health workers and infant mortality

In an East African village, a medical mission operated a "child survival" clinic. The medical missionaries did not make the effort to learn how the people in that particular village understood the medical work that they did. Instead, they believed that the health and survival of children, as an expression of God's concern for human life, was a universal value that every culture would appreciate.

But the villagers did not esteem the work of the mission as highly as the medical personnel expected they would. The villagers affirmed they had a high view of human life, but they seemed indifferent to the high rate of infant mortality in their community. This affirmation for human life and indifference toward infant deaths puzzled the health workers. They saw these two aspects of the host culture as irreconcilable. Even so, the villagers held the two realities together by spiritually interpreting the meaning of infant death. The medical missionaries were unaware of the meanings the villagers placed on infant deaths. Yet these meanings had a profound effect on the work of the mission.

I learned how the villagers interpreted the meaning of the infant deaths while visiting the project. A village resident told me that public health and child survival programs were a waste of time and money. "Why do you say that?" I asked, knowing that particular country had one of the highest infant mortality rates in the world.

"The people who run these projects," my informant told me, "do not understand that village people believe infant deaths are spiritually beneficial. The parents believe that when children die, the infants go to heaven and become mediators for the salvation of their elders.

"Because of this belief, the villagers resist child health programs. Telling them that health programs will help more of their children survive is not necessarily good news. If a mother says she has four living and two deceased children, she is not communicating a tragedy, as the health people believe. She is telling them how many children will continue her heritage, and how many will advocate her salvation."

The health workers had made a serious contextual error. They assumed that they could communicate their cultural values to the villagers, at least regarding infant mortality, without understanding the particular world views of those people. Apparently, the medical personnel gave little thought to the meaning the village residents attached to these deaths.

Unlike the villagers, the health workers did not perceive the tragedy of infant deaths redemptively. In doing so, they missed an important cultural cue by which to communicate the gospel. If the medical personnel had asked the villagers about the high number of infant deaths, or their beliefs concerning them, they would have gained a critical insight into contextualizing the gospel in that culture.

This example makes a good redemptive analogy, one that leads to an opportunity to contextualize the gospel effectively. The people could have transformed their belief that deceased infants advocate salvation for their parents by learning about Christ as the advocate for salvation.

If every culture had analogies that present themselves as well, contextualization would be much simpler. However, redemptive analogies are not always so neat, and contextualizing development work can get cumbersome.

The orchard, the curse, and the thief

In another village, an orchard owner hired a sorcerer to put a fence, in the form of a curse, around his orchard. If intruders penetrated this spiritual fence and entered the orchard, they would be killed instantly.

Everyone in the village had a story to tell about the effectiveness of the curse. The story I heard was about a man who entered the orchard one night, reached for some fruit, and became immobilized. The next day, people found his body frozen in the position in which he died. Both feet were firmly placed on the ground and his fingers gripped the tempting piece of fruit. After that, no other villagers dared to enter the field.

How does Christianity address the curse? Is there a spiritual dynamic, such as a power encounter, within Christianity that confronts its power? Or does Christianity speak prophetically to the curse with a different ethic? Does it transform the destructive power of the curse with the redemptive power of God, as symbolized by *shalom*? Does the Christian ethic say: If a person takes one piece of fruit from your orchard, give him two pieces?

The primal, Western and holistic world views take different approaches to solving the problem. From the perspective of a primal world view, which focuses on power, Christians are likely to support a power encounter. In this situation, the power of Christianity would most likely be used to break the existing curse on the orchard.

Christian ethics that grow out of a modern world view will support, at least theoretically, taking the higher moral road by giving the thief two pieces of fruit. It declares that a person's life is worth more than a piece of fruit.

A holistic perspective strives to create harmony in the village economy. It suggests a redemptive solution to the problem, a solution that focuses on reconciliation instead of a display of power.

Holism suggests that thieves should work for their keep, not only for their good, but for the good of the community. Holism employs the ethics that Paul used when he advised the Ephesians: "He who has been stealing must steal no longer, but must work, doing something useful with his own hands, that he may have something to share with those in need" (Eph. 4:28).

Why contextualization?

The preceding stories illustrate the problems confronting missionaries who attempt to do holistic development work in primal cultures. These situations raise ambiguities for both the cultural hosts and the missionary guests as they seek to integrate Christianity into the host culture.

Addressing these situations and clearing the ambiguities causes many indigenous and foreign missionaries to be less supportive of contextualization. They believe contextualization makes too many concessions to non-Christian religions and cultures.

Other people see contextualization as the key to communicating the gospel cross-culturally. They argue that if we do not contextualize development, it becomes vulnerable to portraying God as irrelevant cultural baggage, a "superfluous, ideological superstructure."[1]

This chapter assumes contextualization has a role in Christian missions because the gospel has to be communicated in some cultural package. It will define the role of contextualization in Christian missions, and examine some problems that occur when we export technological innovations from modern cultures to primal cultures. I will conclude the chapter by applying the principles of critical contextualization to specific missiological situations.

To a large degree, the current support for contextualization is a reaction against non-contextualized mission efforts, particularly efforts from the early stages of the modern mission era. When the early missionaries worked in primal cultures, they assumed Christianity and Western-ization comprised a single, unified package. With few exceptions, these missionaries believed indigenous cultures contained nothing they could use to communicate the Christian message.

So Christians, like the Greeks and Romans who believed other people were barbarians, believed indigenous cultures were irredeemable. They had little doubt that the Christian West was superior to other cultures. This belief was so fundamental to missions that it "operated mainly on an unconscious, presuppositional level."[2] David Barrett quotes Jomo Kenyatta, the first president of Kenya, who wrote: "The Europeans based their assumptions on the conviction that everything that the Africans did or thought was evil."[3]

Western Christians believed that indigenous cultures contributed nothing to Christian worship. Civilizing and Christianizing became the articulated and assumed slogan of most mission agencies. This led one missionary to write in 1844: "No [one] can become a Christian in the true sense of the term, however savage [he] may have been before, without becoming a civilized [person]."[4] Civilization was synonymous with West-ernization.

The ethnocentric beliefs of early missionaries played a significant role in separating indigenous Christians from their cultures. These attitudes highlight the need for modern missionaries to contextualize the gospel. Now, missionaries are no longer so willing to believe that indigenous cultures are beyond redemption. Instead, they believe that all cultures have some aspects that are sinful, some that are redeemable, and some that are spiritually neutral.

Contextualization addresses the spirituality of indigenous cultural forms by incorporating them into worship, or giving them new meaning. In this effort, the missionaries' task changed from one of bringing God to an indigenous culture to identifying God within those cultures. A tribute to one missionary, who seems to have become a legend, was: "You did not bring God to this culture, but led us to realize that he was already among us."

Defining contextualization

The best definition of contextualization that I have read is from *Holistic Evangelism* by Mikha Joedhiswara, a pastor from Indonesia. He defined contextualization as:

> . . . the capacity to respond meaningfully to the gospel within the framework of one's own situation. It is the process by which a local community integrates the gospel message with the real-life context, blending text and context into that single, God-intended

reality called Christian living . . . Contextualization . . . takes into
account the process of secularity, technology and the struggle for
human justice . . .[5]

If we think of world views as maps of our basic assumptions of
reality, contextualization means packaging the gospel to speak to those
assumptions. Contextualization begins with the assumptions people
make, and attempts to understand how the gospel transforms their lives
and cultures, enabling them to worship effectively in their cultures.

Yet contextualization is not static. It begins where people are, and
it transforms them into what God wants them to be. In this sense, *contextualization* and *transformation* are one dynamic.[6] To the Athenians, Paul
communicated the Good News of the God who created the universe, in
the package of the unknown god in the Greek pantheon. In doing so, he
motivated some people to open the package of his message to learn more
about this God.

When Christians from Western cultures communicate the gospel
to people from non-Western cultures, all too often they present the gospel
as dualistic, introducing dualism to a culture where the concept does not
exist. Pius Wakatama shares an illustrative story:

> One day I talked to an angry African Christian leader. As a prin-
> cipal of a Bible school in Africa, he saw the need to provide pro-
> tein for his students. He bought some chickens which the
> students were happy to take care of . . . The hope was that some
> day the chickens would provide meat for the dining table . . .
> When [the] African Christian leader was on study leave, an
> American missionary . . . sold the chickens. To him it was ludi-
> crous for a Bible school to raise chickens.[7]

When Professor B. Makhathini of the University of Swaziland
reflected on the package that brought Christianity to his culture, he said:

> Before the bread of life (the Christian faith) came to our part of
> Africa, it stayed in Europe for over a thousand years. There the
> Europeans added a plastic bag (their own customs) to the bread.
> And when they came to Southern Africa, they fed us the bag
> along with the bread. Now, the plastic bag is making us sick! The
> plastic is theirs. We know that God planned for us to receive the
> bread just as he planned for them to receive it. We can remove
> the plastic, and enjoy the bread.[8]

Perceiving contextualization as packaging is useful in implementing holistic Christian development because it raises questions of *why*

instead of *how*. It focuses on motives, realizing that motives, not methods, address cultural values and behaviors.

Let's think of our houses as the packages we live in, our clothing as the packages we wear, and our vehicles as our transportation packages. If we asked people how they live in their houses, how they wear certain styles of clothing, or how they travel in one type of vehicle or another, we would receive functional answers that would be of little use in knowing who they are.

Useful answers come from why questions. By asking why, we begin to understand, among other things, why people view reality as they do, why they make particular decisions, and why our efforts to relate to them fail or succeed. With why questions we can also focus on transforming values, the bridges between behavior and faith.

The health workers in the African village missed a crucial perception because they did not ask why questions or give the villagers a reason why infant mortality should be reduced. Instead, they assumed the reasons for their work were obvious and they jumped to implementation, the second step of the project. They assumed the community residents shared their values and wanted to learn how to reduce their infant mortality rate.

Unfortunately, the villagers did not share the values of the health workers. If the villagers had understood that child survival is important because life is sacred and that God has provided an advocate for their salvation, they would have had a better appreciation for the benefits of the project. They were not so concerned about how to reduce infant mortality; they needed to know why it should be reduced. To the villagers, their local religion provided an adequate explanation for the role of infant deaths. If the health workers wanted their project to have an impact, they should have addressed the local religious conviction. The project personnel needed to consider this question: How do we package the Good News to people in this culture?

The problem of contextualizing development

Transforming or incorporating indigenous cultural forms in worship is a great step in communicating the gospel cross-culturally. Yet our tendency not to contextualize development projects makes us vulnerable to reversing the progress already made in contextualizing other areas of missions.

The basic problem of contextualizing development is a result of our work's unavoidable dependency on western technological innovations. In many situations, the technological innovations that are a part of development work have displaced traditional practices. Medical programs have replaced traditional healing remedies, and modern pharmaceuticals have replaced ceremonies. Modern agricultural programs with their scientific methods have replaced traditional agricultural rites.

As agents of this transition from tradition to modernity, Christian development workers must ask if technology moves people closer to the kingdom of God or communicates "the triumph of science over religion."[9] We find the answer to this question in the effect technology has on indigenous cultures. Does technology secularize the culture or does it communicate that God is the impetus behind technological progress? The answer can be "yes" to either question, depending on how we communicate the relationship between God and technology.

Christians with a Western world view take technology for granted. In this world view, there is nothing mysterious about computers, fax machines, or antibiotics. We base the operation of these items on scientific principles that we can explain apart from a spiritual or mysterious basis. This leads people to believe and communicate the idea that God, somehow, works in a different sphere of reality.

When Christians bring technological artifacts into primal cultures, the assumption that fax machines, computers, or tape recorders do not have a spiritual basis does not transfer well. The indigenous people, unlike Westerners, may not make such a casual relationship between the power of God and the power of technology. In cultures where the unseen world explains the seen world, the people assume that technology has a spiritual basis. In the primal world view, the God of the missionaries must be responsible in some direct way for the technology the missionaries use.

A friend from a rural village in Chad illustrated this point for me. He told me that the village people see computers, modern medicine, and fax machines as modern expressions of sorcery. "The villagers believe that people from developed cultures," my friend said, "use their spiritual power for good things, whereas the native people use spiritual power in other ways.

"If village sorcerers accept Christianity," he continued, "the village residents believe they can transform their sorcery to more constructive uses. They think that spells, witchcraft and sorcery will be transformed into medicine, fax machines and computers."

Is this belief valid? Can spells, witchcraft and sorcery be transformed into medicine, fax machines and computers? Does technology have a spirit? How should Christians address this belief?

Our approach to these delicate issues is critical for contextualizing Christian development holistically. A major principle of communication is that we cannot avoid communicating. By using computers, fax machines and modern medicine in holistic Christian development, we make a statement about the relationship between the power of God and the power of technology.

What do we want this statement to be? Many who have studied the effects of development on societies suggest that Christian missions make a statement that secularizes cultures by undercutting the spirituality of those cultures. To apply Peter Berger's assessment of modernization to development, development cuts the umbilical cord connecting heaven and earth, creating a lonely, secularized world where only the rumor of God prevails.

Berger's observation complements the concerns of Lesslie Newbigin, who wondered whether the church could convert the Western world. Newbigin saw Christian missionaries as one of the greatest secularizing forces in history. The results of their efforts frequently affirm Rudolph Bultmann's belief that "one cannot use electric lights and radio and call upon modern medicine in case of illness, and at the same time believe in the world of spirits and miracles."[10]

Technology as a product of a religion instead of a culture

Can we affirm that technology grew from the presuppositions of Christianity rather than Western culture? The answer to this question settles the conflict apparent in Western cultures between the existence of God and the power of technology. The conflict has a profound effect on Christian missions and can be mediated through effective contextualization.

Mediating the apparent conflict between science and religion helps us see that science and religion have two distinct purposes. Some theologians believe that science asks the how questions and religion asks the why questions.

This how and why distinction is inadequate; science and religion ask different types of why questions. Science, the systematic pursuit of knowledge, observes relationships between events and proposes explanations for these relationships. It focuses on observing why relationships between created matter develop and form but, in its purest form, science does not apply meaning to these relationships. Diogenes Allen wrote: "The existence of the universe and its basic constituents are taken for granted by our sciences. Scientific laws and theories concern only the transformations of everything that now is."[11]

To the extent that they address different why questions, science and religion are not dichotomous or competitive. Instead, science serves religion by focusing on the intermediate why questions. The answers to these intermediate questions shed light on the ultimate why questions.

Science, for example, can answer why water freezes under some conditions and not under others. It also can measure, predict, and replicate the conditions that cause water to freeze, and explain why water expands when frozen while other chemicals contract. But science does not assign meaning and purpose to this process.

Meaning is a religious concern. Allen argues eloquently that science is a product of Christian faith. His reason for this belief is the Christian conviction that the universe functions in an orderly manner because it depends on a perfect being for its existence. This conviction gives authority to natural observations; they point toward, and symbolize, the Creator who made them possible.

Allen writes that the Greeks, who gave more authority to human thought than to natural observation, did not recognize this hallmark of modern science.[12] Even Aristotle, who respected observed fact, did not recognize the authority it held.[13] So Aristotle missed the religious premises that undergird science.

The second step in mediating the apparent conflict between science and religion is recognizing our fallacious tendency to see Western culture as the source of science. While this fallacy generally goes unchallenged, its opposite is true. Christianity, as Herbert Butterfield, Diogenes Allen and other writers have pointed out, was the impetus that gave birth to science. Natural law, on which we base science, is not an argument against the reality of God. Instead, it is "an expression of the immutable faithfulness of the Creator, who has made life possible by establishing a constant order of nature."[14]

Shalom for the shamans

If we returned to an earlier question asking whether technology has a spirit, the answer, in a broad sense, is yes. Since Christians do not believe the world is a closed system, they cannot affirm that the laws of science and the power of technology are self-perpetuating. Therefore, the scientific discoveries and technological innovations that form the basis for these laws and powers are made possible, if not guided, by the Creator. In this sense, God, the Creator, is the spirit of, or behind, technology.

If we go back to another previous question, we can ask whether modern technology will replace spells, curses and witchcraft if the shamans who perform these functions convert to Christianity. If we contextualize development holistically, modern technology will not replace the spells, curses and witchcraft. Instead, the perception of power that makes spells, witchcraft and sorcery possible will undergo transformation to enable the shamans to see God's redemptive power in their communities. They will see that the power of God is of a different nature, not simply a stronger power. God does not simply inspire them to get more of what they have, but transforms the power they already have.

If the shamans convert to Christianity, their spiritual powers, as the villagers expect, will be transformed to do good things as God's will is revealed and understood. They will use the power of Christ to heal the sick, bring comfort to the oppressed, and render justice to the poor. They will observe God working through nature, technology, and other physical media to bring *shalom*.

Implementing contextualization

A major problem of implementing contextualization is believing the either-or principle of cultures. In the early years of Christian missions, Western Christians thought the cultural practices of the indigenous people were uniformly bad. Now the pendulum is swinging to depict indigenous cultural practices as uniformly good and redeemable.

One extreme is just as problematic as the other. All cultures have practices that can be redeemed and ones that must be discarded. The problems include deciding which practices to redeem or eliminate, who makes the decisions, and establishing the criteria to guide the decisions.

Paul Hiebert's thoughts on critical contextualization shed some light on this dilemma. While solving the problem of communicating the gospel as absolute truth through culturally relative media, he developed four principles of contextualization from the work of Jacob Loewen and John Geertz. These principles are: 1) understand what the people believe about the problem; 2) create a bridge between Scripture and the problem; 3) the people evaluate their customs in light of Scripture; and 4) practice the contextualized ethic.[15]

I am going to apply these principles to a variety of missiological contexts. I will use a health education example to illustrate how the principles of critical contextualization solve an existing missions problem. The second example, about an agronomist telling a farmer that spirits will destroy the farmland, illustrates how critical contextualization can prevent future problems. The third example analyzes the use of an electroshock machine and explains how we extend existing beliefs so that they can become more holistic. I give the fourth example, deciding whether to exorcise blood in a mission hospital, to show the dynamic nature of critical contextualization. It shows that the effectiveness of a solution at one place in time will fade as cultures change.

Health education and the will of Allah

Mary, my wife, developed a health education curriculum in a folk Islamic culture to teach mothers of infants whose children were suffering from nutrition-related illnesses. In these lessons, she stressed the importance of personal hygiene and good nutrition in maintaining the health of children. She emphasized that mothers should be aware of the germs that cause illnesses, and feed children food that contains nutrients that contribute to the well-being of the children.

Mary's lessons were good recipes for health, but they had a limited effect because the mothers did not understand nutrients and germs. Germs could not be seen, and the people had little trust in the technology that makes them visible. In the mothers' world view, non-Muslims who did not submit to Allah's will used germs and nutrients to explain things that were obviously the will of Allah.

This tension between submitting to Allah's will and applying the teachings of a non-Muslim emerged one day after Mary taught a class on the causes of diarrhea. She concluded the lesson by asking the women why their children get infected with the disease. Mary expected the women to reflect upon the material she had just taught. She wanted to hear answers such as, "The water my children drink contains germs. If I do not boil or bleach it before the children drink it, they will get diarrhea." Instead, an articulate woman exclaimed, "My baby has diarrhea because Allah sends it!"

The woman spoke for the entire class, and expressed a fundamental failure in the lessons. The lessons did not address the spiritual dilemma the mothers experienced. The lessons gave them no basis for reconciling the existence of germs with the sovereignty of Allah. If children suffered from diarrhea, Allah was responsible. What else could the mothers believe? Even if their world view had room for germs, germs could not change the will of Allah. Allah is the final explanation for everything.

Contextualizing health education

We can reduce the problem of contextualizing the gospel in general, and development in particular by asking: How do we hold the benevolent sovereignty of God and the destructive existence of germs together to affirm the truth of both statements? The principles of critical contextualization contribute to solving this problem.

Principle #1: Understand what the people believe about the problem.

To contextualize the gospel critically, we must first analyze the culture to learn how the people perceive the problem. From the perspective of a modern theistic world view, fatalism was the problem in the project where my wife worked. For the women, the problem was accepting the sovereignty of Allah. The women's presence in the class showed their willingness to accept help, but the class did not address their basic problem in a way that made sense to them. How could they reconcile Allah's will with the presence of germs and this health information? The mothers were powerless to reconcile these two opposing choices.

Principle #2: Create a bridge between Scripture and the problem.

The second step of critical contextualization is to examine the Scriptures and create a bridge between Scripture and the problem at hand. How can we apply scriptural teachings on illness and the sovereignty of God to the women's dilemma?

The Scriptures acknowledge that people get sick and teach that God, in his sovereignty, heals the sick through various means. The Scriptures also teach that good nutrition and hygiene are important to maintaining good health. Major portions of the books of Moses contain laws that protect the health of the Hebrew community. They include many regulations regarding health, cleanliness, and diets.

Can we apply these laws to the Muslim community? Definitely! The Muslims recognize the *Torah* as the book of the prophet Muuse (Moses). Through the *Torah*, the mothers can see Muuse's concern for the health of his people, mirroring their concern for the health of their children.

Considering the Islamic view of God's sovereignty, and the common heritage that Hebrews, Christians, and Muslims share, a more appropriate question than asking the mothers why their children are sick is: What did the Prophet Moses say about illness?

Principle #3: The people evaluate their customs in light of Scripture.

The third step of critical contextualization is to enable the people to evaluate their customs in light of biblical teaching. Do they believe that Allah, in his sovereignty, gives them the freedom to make decisions? Can their faith in a sovereign God be transformed to incorporate human responsibility?

For the women at the project, this step would empower them to see how Allah reveals his will as they make decisions every day to enhance their own and their families' welfare. They do not sit passively waiting for Allah to gather firewood, deliver water, cook food, feed the livestock, and tend the garden. The very thought is blasphemous. The decisions they make in each activity reveal their freedom, in the will of God, to effect change in their environments.

Principle #4: Practice the contextualized ethic.

The fourth step is to practice a new contextualized ethic. In my wife's project, the women empowered themselves to care for the health of their children by accepting this responsibility in submission to Allah.

A handy teaching tool for communicating the values of cleanliness, hygiene, and immunizations was the analogy of a fence. People build a fence around a garden to keep animals out. Cleanliness, hygiene, and immunizations work like fences that we build around our bodies to keep germs out.

Without a flashlight, we cannot see the animals that invade our garden at night. When we wake up the next day, we know they were there when we see the damage they caused. By using a flashlight we can see the animals and minimize the damage they may cause. In the same way, we cannot see germs without using a microscope, but we know they are present when our children get sick.

Flashlights and microscopes are different expressions of the technology we use to fulfill the responsibility God gave us to protect ourselves and our environments from damage and illness. We use proper health care to protect our bodies from germs, just as we build fences to protect our gardens from intruders.

A Christian development agency practiced a contextualized ethic differently in a health education project similar to the one Mary developed. They asked a respected local spiritual leader to endorse the health lessons. This endorsement gave the people the security that the material from foreigners was not offensive to their faith. They accepted the reality of germs, and gained a new understanding of how God works in the universe.

This understanding was a first step in bringing them closer to the kingdom of God. They saw how God cares for them by including in his Word the laws that protect their health and welfare. The contextualized ethic brought *shalom* to their community by showing how God works redemptively in the situations that threaten their lives and their well-being.

Do the spirits destroy the land?

In an African village, an agronomist met a farmer who was burning debris on his field. The farmer had only manual tools, and he found that slashing and burning the debris was a quick and easy way of clearing the fields.

The agronomist told the farmer that fire destroys the nutrients in the soil. "During the next few decades," the agronomist continued instructing the farmer, "the farmland will turn to a desert if farmers continue to burn their fields." The agronomist advised the farmer to rake the debris into compost pits, and told the farmer about the benefits and techniques of composting.

The agronomist helped the farmer compare the benefits of composting to the consequences of burning by focusing on the need to build nutrients in the soil. After the conversation, the agronomist was confident that the farmer would choose to compost, but the farmer had other concerns. "What are nutrients, anyway?" he wondered. "What relationship do they have to the spirits who make the crops grow?"

The agronomist and the farmer were making different assumptions about the environment. Still, this did not deter the agronomist. He confidently told the farmer, "The fires attract the spirits that destroy the nutrients in the soil. These destructive spirits have power over the good spirits that make the land fertile." This logic made sense to the farmer, and he chose composting instead of burning.

The agronomist's statement was apparently effective, but was it justified? Did it effectively communicate humankind's stewardship of creation? Was the farmer empowered to exercise the dominion he has over his land, or was his fear of the spirits reinforced, preventing him from transforming his view of God?

If we applied the principles of critical contextualization to this situation, they would not support the statement that the fire attracts the spirits that destroy the nutrients. Since the agronomist does not believe that the fire attracts the spirits, introducing the idea brings his personal integrity into question and creates a problem for the farmer.

The first principle of critical contextualization is understanding how the people perceive the problem; it does not attempt to interpret the problem for them. The farmer understood that his problem was how to clear his land. In solving his problem, he used a technique that was acceptable within his culture, but one that would eventually destroy the soil. It was easy to lead the farmer to believe his fires would attract destructive spirits that would destroy his land. But he was not making that connection before the conversation with the agronomist.

In creating a bridge between Scripture and the problem (the second principle), we find no evidence in Scripture to support the idea that spirits will destroy the land. Instead, Scripture clearly shows that God gave people dominion over creation, making them responsible for caring for it.[16]

The third principle (the people evaluate their customs in light of Scripture) focuses on what the people believe about their practice of slashing and burning in light of scriptural teaching. The emphasis here is on their roles as stewards of a fragile environment, in service to God. The idea that spirits will destroy the land, while believable, is not a part of their customs. At best, it is a bad and unnecessary solution to a difficult problem.

In the fourth principle (the people practice the contextualized ethic), the people will practice composting instead of burning. They will support this practice since they have a high regard for the land as the handiwork of God.

What is the relationship of the electroshock machine to the spirits?

A few decades ago, a mission clinic that operated in an African village used an electroshock machine to treat depression and anxiety. Apparently, the use of the machine was successful; people in the village frequently requested electroshock therapy, making it the treatment of choice.

When the people receiving this treatment were asked what they understood about it, they said the machine cast out the spirits that cause depression and anxiety. The people were often disappointed if the health workers gave them medicine instead of placing them on the machine. They believed the machine, not the medicine, had the power to cast out the spirits.

How should we explain the effectiveness of the machine and pharmaceuticals to these people? If we applied the principles of critical contextualization to this situation, would they support the people's belief that the machine casts out the spirits of anxiety and depression?

Considering the villagers' world view, an initial examination of the problem using the principles of critical contextualization supports their belief that the machine casts out spirits. Yet the principles extend this belief to teach people to see other causes of depression and anxiety. In this manner, the principles of critical contextualization transform the belief that particular spirits cause all illnesses to include general spiritual causes as well. These general spiritual causes are a result of living in a fallen creation.

The first and second principles of critical contextualization support this conclusion. The people understand that their problem has a spiritual nature. Taken at face value, we can conclude that Scripture supports the idea that spirits can cause depression, anxiety, and other illnesses (see Mark 9, Luke 8 and 13).

If people evaluate their customs in light of Scripture (the third step of critical contextualization), their belief in spirits is not the problem. The problem lies in introducing new technology into their culture. We could lead them to see the curative purpose of the technology as an extension of their belief about curing depression and anxiety by casting out spirits. This extension, however, may be unnecessary. Since the electroshock machine is not a part of their culture, we cannot evaluate it as if it were part of their culture. We must address it as an import to the culture.

The contextualization question, then, asks whether we should affirm the assumption of the villagers that the machine casts out spirits. If the villagers believe spirits cause depression and anxiety, does that mean spirits cause all depression and anxiety? Can we take the opportunity, with the introduction of the machine, to introduce a new understanding of anxiety and depression into the culture?

Critical contextualization affirms the introduction of a new understanding of anxiety and depression into the culture. The theory that we can treat depression and anxiety by sending electrical impulses through the body does not eliminate the possibility that spirits also cause illnesses. Instead, it creates an opportunity to introduce the belief that the fallen state of creation causes illnesses.

The fallen state of creation causes illnesses to have general and particular origins. The nature of both origins is spiritual. The particular origins are spirits; the general origins are the effects of living in a fallen creation. The coexistence of beliefs in the particular and general origins of illnesses is not contradictory. Instead, in their coexistence, these beliefs recognize the physical and spiritual implications of the fallen state of creation. Holistic Christian development works to treat illnesses that result from the general and particular effects of our fallen creation.

Should the pastor exorcise the blood bank of a Christian mission?

In an African village, a Christian missionary medical team has a blood bank. The medical team carefully screens the blood to detect impurities. The medical team's indifference to spiritual impurities concerned the village pastor. He asked the missionaries if any of the blood they used in transfusions came from people who employed sorcery or witchcraft.

The missionaries did not know whether the blood donors used sorcery, and they really didn't care. In their world view, blood is a substance that transports oxygen through the body. Its spiritual significance is symbolic. If the donors used sorcery at some time in their lives, the important properties of the extracted blood did not change.

The pastor remained unconvinced of the validity of the missionaries' view of blood. He saw blood as the medium that transports life, and did not want the villagers to receive blood that may be cursed or contain impure spirits. He wanted to break the power of any curses that existed in the blood the medical missionaries were using in their transfusions.

Should the missionaries allow the pastor to exorcise their blood bank? What statement does permitting or granting this request make to the villagers about the Christian message? What decision communicates the redemptive power of God to bring *shalom* to the community?

In discussing this situation with the pastor, I learned that he and I expressed our spirituality differently. My spirituality, primarily because of my Western world view, was abstract. Therefore, I valued blood for its ability to transport oxygen through my body. To me, blood lacked actual spiritual value apart from affirming God's ability to use it to enable my body to function properly. My concern with receiving blood transfusions was whether the blood had any impurities that would prevent it from fulfilling its function within my body.

The pastor, undoubtedly because of his primal world view, perceived his spirituality more concretely. He believed blood is the medium of spiritual power. While he granted that blood transports oxygen through the body, its ability to transport spiritual power was more important to him. He emphasized how sorcerers and shamans use the blood of animals and people to invoke the powers of the spirits. The pastor reminded me that Christ shed his blood for the forgiveness of sins. "Blood," he reiterated, "has power."

In his world view, if someone did not purify the blood, the spiritual powers of the donors may transfer to the patients who receive it. In this situation, Christians who receive blood would be infected with non-Christian spiritual powers, ironically, through blood provided by a Christian mission.

He asked, "Why can't the missionaries see this obvious problem?"

I explained that people with a Western world view do not believe that Christian or non-Christian spiritual powers inhabit blood. For most Christians from Western cultures, the spiritual power of blood is symbolic. It is a physical substance that communicates a spiritual reality.

"Do demons flee from symbols?" the pastor persisted.

For me, whether demons flee symbols was not central to our discussion. I imagined that symbols were as powerful as the reality behind them. But I had other questions: Does the truth of the Christian message lie in its power to chase demons? Or does Christianity, through the work of the clinic, communicate a greater truth to the villagers? Do the villagers see beyond the power of the blood to grasp the truth of the redemptive work of Christ in all creation? How do the demons fit within the scope of Christ's redemptive work?

Using the principles of critical contextualization could help us answer these questions. If we applied these principles to the problem of exorcising the spirits from the blood, the mission probably would acquiesce to the pastor's desire to exorcise the blood. This need should fade as the community's fear of spirits is transformed when the people come to understand the scope of evil within God's redemptive work.

Critical contextualization and the demons

The first principle of critical contextualization acknowledges the problem as the people understand it. In contrast to the agronomist who introduced spirits into a situation, the spirits in this circumstance pose a current problem. The people believe these spirits are real. For the missionaries, these spirits create a stumbling block that prevents the villagers from using the mission's services.

The scriptural affirmation for the existence of demons addresses the second principle of critical contextualization. For this principle, the initial acceptance of demons is adequate. Discussions about whether demons exist as disembodied spirits or metaphors for particular behaviors are counterproductive. The villagers believed, as the first century Jews apparently did, that demons were autonomous spiritual entities.

In this situation, the third principle of critical contextualization is crucial: the community of the faithful evaluate their customs in light of Scripture. While we may believe that the demons mentioned in Scripture are similar to those encountered in the village, the biblical understanding of demons is probably different from that of the villagers.

The Bible sees evil, and demons that embody evil, within the scope of creation. It does not imply that God created evil, but it implies that evil grew out of creation. The biblical view of creation does not support a dualism between good and evil, depicting the autonomous existence of evil threatening the sovereignty of God. Instead, the Bible teaches that evil is perverted good. Evil is a rebellion against the good nature of the Creator. God saw all creation, and said it was good (Gen. 1:31). In the Fall, the goodness of creation suffered from the consequences of sin, causing it to fall short of the goodness with which God created it.

Considering the third principle and the biblical teaching on the goodness of creation, we can see the demons as evil, but within the context of good. While demons have the choice to rebel and pervert their goodness, they do not have the power to pervert God's goodness. Because of God's power the villagers who participate in God's redemptive work in creation do not have to live in fear of the spirits. They can now live in faith knowing that the evil the spirits may provoke is subject to the goodness of God.

The fourth principle of critical contextualization is practicing the contextualized ethic. Since critical contextualization is dynamic, the present position of the villagers will not be their final position. As a first generation of converts from animism, they are making a transition between their fear of spirits and their faith in God. This transition will continue over generations. Eventually, they will view their fear of spirits in the context of God's sovereignty and they will evaluate the need to exorcise them accordingly.

The integrity and relevancy of the gospel

We cannot undervalue contextualization when we bring the gospel to cultures where the people's main concerns are having advocates for salvation, the protection of people and livelihoods from curses, or receiving blood affected by sorcery. Contextualization answers questions that make the gospel relevant to the particular concerns of people in various cultures.

Critical contextualization transforms the packages of any particular culture to maintain the integrity of the gospel and its ability to be relevant in that culture. As the examples in this chapter show, critical contextualization provides a good test for evaluating the validity of contextualizing the gospel, particularly in the relationship of the gospel to development.

The principles of critical contextualization do not affirm every cultural practice, but they enable local Christian communities to evaluate their cultural practices in light of Christian teaching. Local communities can decide how to package the gospel in a way that makes sense to them without compromising its teachings and principles.

In Western cultures and cultures affected by Westernization, the package will undergo a transformation from dualism to holism. In primal cultures, contextualization transforms the people's perception that they are at the mercy of the spirits and enables them to see God working redemptively to perfect their faith.

NOTES

1. Karl Heim, "Christian Faith and the Growing Power of Secularism," *Religion and Culture*, Walter Liebrecht, ed. (Harper & Row, 1959), p. 188.

2. David J. Bosch, *Transforming Mission: Paradigm Shifts in Theology of Mission* (Maryknoll: Orbis Books, 1991), p. 292.

3. David B. Barrett, *Schism & Renewal in Africa: An Analysis of Six Thousand Contemporary Religious Movements* (New York: Oxford University Press, 1968), p. 86. (The statement is from: Jomo Kenyatta, *Facing Mt. Kenya* (London: Secker and Warburg, 1938).

4. Jon Bonk, "'All Things to All People'—The Missionary as a Racist-Imperialist, 1860-1918," *Missiology: An International Review*, Vol. 8:3 (July 1980): 302.

5. Mikha Joedhiswara "Holistic Evangelism: On Suffering in the Face of Overwhelming Poverty and Multifaceted Religiosity," *Mission Focus*, Vol. 20:2 (June 1992): 32-33.

6. From personal correspondence with Paul G. Hiebert, April 1992.

7. Pius Wakatama, *Independence for the Third World Church: An African's Perspective on Missionary Work* (Downers Grove: InterVarsity Press, 1978), pp. 52-53.

8. K. P. Yohannan, *Why the World Waits: Exposing the Reality of Modern Missions* (Lake Mary, Florida: Creation House Publishers, 1991) p. 103.

9. Paul G. Hiebert, "Critical Contextualization," *International Bulletin of Missionary Research,* (July 1987), 11(3): 105.

10. Lesslie M. Newbigin, "Can the West Be Converted?" *International Bulletin of Missionary Research,* (January 1987), 11:1: 2-7.

11. Diogenes Allen, *Christianity in a Post Modern World: The Full Wealth of Conviction* (Louisville: Westminster/John Knox Press, 1989), p. 53.

12. Ibid., p. 25.

13. Ibid.

14. Heim, p. 189.

15. Paul G. Hiebert, "Critical Contextualization," *International Bulletin of Missionary Research* (July 1987): 109.

16. While the argument can be made that keeping the spirits away from the land is caring for the land, the focus of Scripture is giving humankind responsibility to care for creation.

FOUR

Management:
Facilitating God's redemptive power

Once when we were going to the place of prayer,
we were met by a slave girl who had a spirit
by which she predicted the future.
She earned a great deal of money
for her owners by fortune-telling.
This girl followed Paul and the rest of us, shouting,
"These men are servants of the Most High God,
who are telling you the way to be saved."
She kept this up for many days.
Finally Paul became so troubled
that he turned around and said to the spirit,
"In the name of Jesus Christ
I command you to come out of her!"
At that moment the spirit left her.
Acts 16:16-18

HAVE YOU EVER thought of Paul's confrontation with this slave girl as a management problem? Luke's narrative tells us the girl was noted for telling fortunes. She declared to the community that Paul and his associates were servants of the Most High God, proclaiming the way to salvation. Should Paul accept the message for the truth it contains, or evaluate the message on the ethos of the person who delivered it? Is truth, despite the messenger, still truth?

In the scheme of the physical-spiritual dichotomy, Paul's confrontation with this slave girl is a spiritual problem. The spirit, as Figure 4.1[1] on page 72 illustrates, is in the upper tier of the universe. To cast the spirit from the girl, Paul must invoke the good spiritual powers (God or angels) to defeat an evil spiritual power (the demons), particularly the

Figure 4.1   Western world view   Figure 4.2   Holistic world view

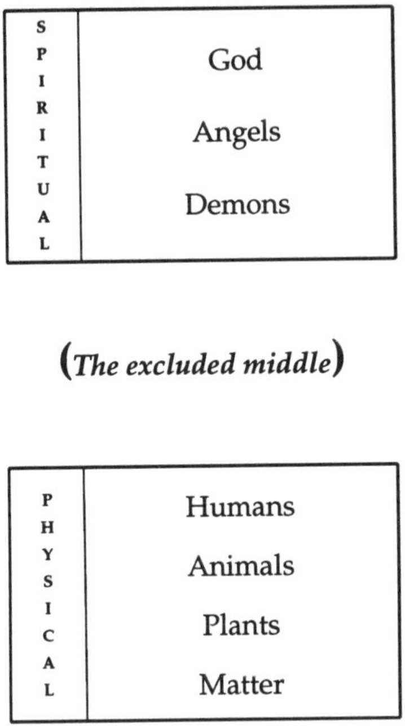

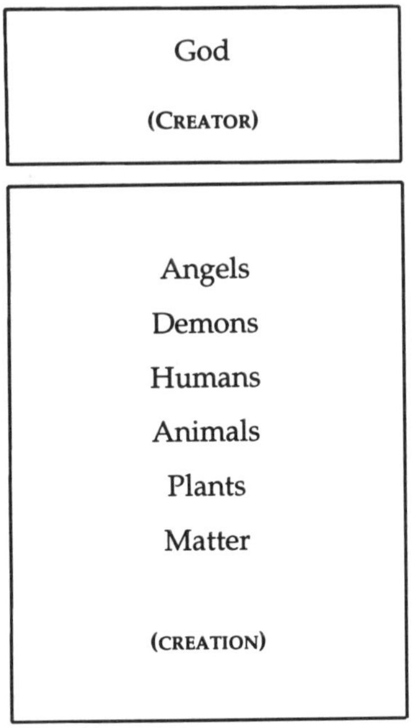

	God
S P I R I T U A L	Angels
	Demons

(The excluded middle)

	Humans
P H Y S I C A L	Animals
	Plants
	Matter

God

(CREATOR)

Angels

Demons

Humans

Animals

Plants

Matter

(CREATION)

one that spoke through this girl. In the scheme of Figure 4.1, no management decision is necessary. The nature of the spirits is clear, and management remains a mundane issue in the lower realms of creation.

But the way Paul dealt with the girl and the spirit that was influencing her leads us to believe Figure 4.1 presents reality as less ambigu-
ous than it is. If Figure 4.1 was an accurate reflection of reality, Paul
would not have a management problem. The spirit, because of its evil
nature, would unquestionably be cast from the girl. Yet Paul waited several days before he made a decision regarding the girl. Apparently, Paul
gave some thought to reconciling the truth of the girl's statement with the
nature of the spirit that was influencing her. Perhaps Paul, in this situation and in others (1 Cor. 5:13; 1 Tim. 1:20), saw the possibility of managing evil for the sake of good.

Figure 4.2, which illustrates a creation that is reconciled to God,
gives a more accurate portrayal of the problem Paul faced. This model
shows that Paul saw the demon as a fallen element of creation that
embodied itself in the girl. It also has room for Paul to see the demon as a
label for the girl's behavior. In either situation, Paul's efforts worked
toward managing created elements redemptively.

Paul and the decision-making cycle

Decisions like Paul's frequently confront Christians who are managing development holistically. They are not easy decisions to make. Let's imagine what went through Paul's mind as the woman followed him. If he thought like a management theorist, he went through the steps in the following cycle.

Paul's first step was to identify the problem (see Figure 4.3). He had to separate the truth of the message from the nature of the messenger. His concern was whether he should solve the problem by letting the truth speak for itself, or whether the nature of the messenger—the spirit—would insult the integrity of the message. The management question is whether truth, despite its source, is still truth.

The second step of Paul's management decision was examining the environment that perpetuated the problem. Evidently, the woman had credibility in the community and she earned a great deal of money for her owners by telling fortunes. Will the community believe her message because they believe her fortunes?

If Paul examines the impact of the problem on the community, he will see that it has profound implications as the people receive the Christian message. If the people believe the message because they believe the fortunes the girl tells them, they probably won't see any difference between the gospel and the fortunes. Instead of seeing the uniqueness of the gospel, they could associate it with one of the many messages that the

Figure 4.3   Management decision-making cycle

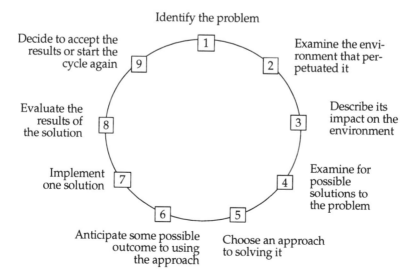

spirit in the girl communicated to them. This makes the girl an annoyance that will hinder Paul's work.

Paul's possible solutions included: 1) passively accepting the girl's role in announcing the identities of Paul and his team; 2) integrating her into the team; or 3) casting the demon from her. The third solution would end her message and the attendant publicity.

Anticipating the results of each solution sheds some light on the choices Paul faced. If Paul passively assented to the girl's presence and her message, he could benefit from the decision of waiting to see how the community would respond. If the girl became an annoyance, he could cast the demon out of her. Otherwise, she might attract a following in the community. The possibility of incorporating her into the team had serious problems. It was the least desirable of the three solutions.

After three days, Paul implemented one solution by choosing to cast the demon from the girl. Apparently, he made a good decision. Paul and his team accepted the results instead of starting the cycle a second time. Luke does not mention her again.

Management and holistic Christian development

In this chapter we will look at similar problems that confront people who are managing Christian development holistically. We will see that management occurs in both Western and primal cultures, but both cultures perceive it differently.

In Western cultures, management is an art we can place on either side of the physical-spiritual dichotomy. It all depends on the nature of the material being managed and the values of the managers. It is an area that Christians in the West want to spiritualize—or sanctify—by developing principles to define management that is uniquely Christian. In primal cultures, management takes a different form. It is more passive, causing people to respond or submit to the whims of the unseen world.

A problem confronted me a few days after I became the manager of a development project in a folk Islamic culture. Someone stole a large sum of traveler's checks from the room where my family was temporarily living. I informed a few staff members about the loss and they did not show surprise. They told me a staff member named Sarah took the money.

"How do you know Sarah took the money?" I asked.

"Because she has a *jinn* [a spirit, good or bad],"[2] came the response.

"How do you know she has a *jinn*?" I inquired.

"Because money has been taken before. The last time it happened, the previous manager hired a sheikh to find out who did it. He lined every staff member up, looked into our eyes, and saw a *jinn* in Sarah. We concluded the *jinn* in Sarah caused her to steal the money."

"Did anyone else see the *jinn*?" I asked.

"No one else can see it," they continued. "The sheikh has double sight. He can see physical and spiritual things. The rest of us can see only physical things."

"Why didn't you relieve Sarah of her job?" I asked. (For them, the question was culturally irrelevant: Why fire Sarah for behavior that was caused by a *jinn*?)

"We do not fire people from jobs in our culture," came the expected reply. "We know that Sarah has a *jinn* so we protect ourselves from her. If we are careful, she (under the influence of her *jinn*) will not hurt us."

I was under obligation to investigate the theft for the Western agency I worked for, and found myself caught between two worlds. I had lived in the local culture long enough to know the staff's commitment to the integrity of their explanation. But my North American agency required an investigation that would produce as much verifiable data as possible.

During the next few days, I investigated the theft according to standard Western management procedures. After the investigation, I was satisfied that I had come to the right conclusion. I wrote a report that convinced its readers beyond a reasonable doubt that a former staff member, not Sarah, took the money.

Months later, after my family had moved to a permanent house, I was astonished to find the stolen traveler's checks in a desk drawer in our new home. Where did they come from?

I knew we did not misplace them during all those months. My wife and I had moved things in and out of that desk drawer several times to prepare for trips. The checks were not there. Otherwise, we would have found them.

The answer to what I saw as the mysterious return of the checks was obvious to the staff. Sarah went to an exorcist, who cast the *jinn* out of her, and she was free to return the checks. Sarah gave the checks to our housekeeper, who was part of her extended family, to return them to us anonymously.

My investigation did not identify the right person. I facetiously wondered whether I needed double-sight to manage projects in this culture. However, I realized that managing Christian development holistically bridges the gap between the two cultural interpretations of the event.

The *jinn* undoubtedly was part of the environment, but we interpreted its existence differently. The staff members saw an external, disembodied spirit influencing or dictating Sarah's behavior by embodying itself in her. Sarah and the community were powerless to address the *jinn* or her behavior.

In contrast to the community, I saw the spirit as a cultural explanation for behavior the community did not understand or did not want to manage. I was open to the possibility that the community's explanation was valid, but this possibility did not fit into my investigation. In this regard, the *jinn* was not so much an external spirit that embodied itself in Sarah. It was a label, or a metaphor, for Sarah's behavior.

Defining management holistically

If we define management as facilitating an expected outcome in a given environment, managing holistic Christian development is somewhat analogous to blending the experience of driving and sitting in the back of a pick-up truck.

Christians, particularly Westerners, drive the truck. We move into the future at 60 miles per hour, looking ahead, planning the trip, organizing the resources to get there, carrying the passengers along, controlling the speed of the vehicle, and evaluating the progress of the journey. We commit this process to God with the faith that he affirms it.

In primal cultures, such as those of folk Muslims, God (Allah) drives the truck; the people sit in the back. They are backing into the future at 60 miles an hour, depending on God to do the planning, leading, organizing, controlling and evaluating. Allah is responsible for anything that happens. The human responsibility is to submit to Allah's will.

Consider how the environment, when viewed from the driver's seat, contrasts with the view from the back of the truck. The orientation of the people in the driver's seat is toward the future. A rapidly approaching future consumes the present. The people keep their eyes focused several car lengths ahead, constantly alert for emerging obstacles. As the present races by, the future becomes clearer.

The past becomes less important than the future or the present. Occasionally, the drivers glance in the rearview mirror to see what is catching up to them. Periodically, they consult a map to compare the present situation to the past and future. The past and present are viewed— and valued—in relation to the future.

From the back of the truck, the past is the primary focus. Those in the back of the truck cannot see the future.[3] The present is flying into the past, creating an illusion of instability in the present. The instability does not settle until the present moves far enough into the past. If people look far enough down the road, the environment appears stable. They see more clearly as the passing environment gets farther from them.

Holistic Christian management affects primal and modern cultures

Because of these differing perceptions, the management of holistic Christian development takes a different approach in modern and primal cultures, even when it addresses similar issues and problems. It seeks to transform and redeem elements in the environment in both cultures, trying to understand how God works redemptively in each culture.

In primal cultures, holistic Christian development recognizes the validity of indigenous cultural elements—expressed rationally and trans-rationally—such as dreams, ancestors, contemporary and genealogical relationships, and values. Holistic Christian development seeks to facilitate relationships between these elements that can be characterized by *shalom*. This occurs by understanding the intrinsic, transformational or redemptive values of the cultural elements.

In modern cultures, managing Christian development holistically means seeing management as more than a rational or mechanical process. It recognizes the influence of values, spiritual convictions and transrational elements on the management process, realizing that God reveals his will and affirms change in many ways. In this modern world view, we realize *shalom* through the reconciliation of the rational and the non-rational.

Managing medical treatment is characteristic of the managerial differences in primal and modern cultures. In modern cultures, physicians examine symptoms to diagnose illnesses and determine probable causes. They view the human body, as Wade Davis writes,

> . . . essentially as a machine, an exceedingly complex mechanism that can be understood, modified and repaired . . . Physicians work best when they can identify and eliminate disease-causing agents . . . Health is defined in strictly clinical terms by physicians. The fate of the spirit is relegated to religious specialists who have little to say about their followers' physical well-being.[4]

When a physician adequately defines a medical problem, he or she develops a treatment plan to remove the obstacles to the patient's good health. The physician then organizes human and medical resources to deliver treatment efficiently and effectively. He or she controls the input of resources according to the prescribed plan. After a course of treatment, the doctor evaluates the results in relation to anticipated outcomes. Did the treatment do what it was expected to do?

If the treatment's effectiveness is less than optimal, the cycle begins again. The physician redefines the problem and anticipated results. He or she redevelops the treatment plan, and reorganizes human and medical resources. There is a reevaluation of the results of the second course of treatment according to the anticipated outcomes. If the anticipated results do not occur with the second course of treatment, the physician makes an evaluation of the feasibility for a third cycle of treatment.

Holistic Christian development affirms the need for the rational nature of this cycle. Yet it also recognizes that doctors treat people, not illnesses, and it emphasizes the roles of hope, faith and reconciliation in the healing process.

In primal cultures, in contrast to modern ones, the management factors in medical treatment are more transrational. Factored into the treatment are "ideas concerning the spiritual realm, mind-body interactions, the interplay among humanity, the environment and the cosmos."[5] These factors include mythological, historical and contemporary influences such as ancestors, spirits, genealogies and religious figures.

Kivuto Ndeti writes about the treatment of a girl whom physicians initially diagnosed and treated as having cerebral malaria.[6] The girl's parents brought her to a traditional medical practitioner (TMP) after they believed the physicians' treatment proved ineffective. This TMP initially managed the treatment by examining the girl's genealogy along her paternal and maternal lines. He discovered that the girl's maternal ancestors suffered from the same illness. The impersonal management of modern medical treatment would have diagnosed the illness as genetic. Yet the TMP saw the illness relationally.

The TMP's treatment plan included a ceremony to appease the ancestors. The resources he organized and controlled included a goat and some herbs. He rubbed the blood from the sacrificed goat on the girl's eyes; he mixed the herbs with the goat's meat, which he then cooked and ate. The final step of the treatment was arranging a traditional dance.

After an evaluation of the results of the treatment, they found the girl had been cured. Apparently, she experienced healing through a catharsis that brought a sense of unity between her, her environment and the spiritual powers.

This type of situation challenges people who are managing Christian development holistically to consider a redemptive response to the influence of mythological, contemporary and historical relationships. The management task is to understand how cultural values, mythology, and genealogical or contemporary figures in a particular culture point toward the redemptive and transformational role of Christ. More specifically, it tries to find how the blood of Christ, our spiritual ancestor, and not the blood of goats, plays a role in managing change.

Understanding the environment of primal cultures

When we perceive the management of Christian development

holistically, the management task becomes understanding how to address the elements in the environment to reflect God's redemptive power.

As previously indicated, the elements of the environment differ in primal and modern cultures. Ancestors play an important role in the managerial environment of primal cultures. They are frequently perceived as the living dead who serve as mediators between God and humankind. A person's genealogy and cultural values are also vital factors in the decisions he or she makes to implement change in primal cultures.

The managerial environment of modern cultures, in contrast to primal cultures, depends more on empirically verified elements. Since holistic development practitioners are more likely to confront, and misunderstand, the non-empirical elements of primal cultures, this section of the chapter will focus on understanding these elements.

Ancestors

When managers from modern cultures find themselves working with people who need to relate to their ancestors, the managers feel that these people are living in the past. But these people are not living in the past. They are bringing their ancestors forward—the ancestors are "eternally present."

Ancestors influence many decisions, and this influence is generally conservative. The living, unwilling to provoke the anger and jealousy of the ancestors, resist making decisions their ancestors would not have made. Farmers in one African village would not use new agricultural methods or plant new vegetables because they did not have the peace that comes with the ancestors' approval. In another village, a family would not live in a new house because it was better than the houses their ancestors lived in. They did not dare to provoke the jealousy of their ancestors.

In a third village, one in the southern hemisphere, agriculturalists proved that planting corn in September instead of December would result in a 60 percent greater yield. Each year the villagers agreed that planting would begin in September during the following year, but each year they did not plant until December. After hours of discussion, the agriculturalists finally learned the villagers' problem: the ancestors would not give permission to plant before December. Without permission from the ancestors, the villagers were helpless to change their planting cycles.

Managing ancestral relationships redemptively calls for the reinterpretation of God's redemptive work through our personal and cultural histories. It affirms that God uses history to make his will known. In a refugee camp in Thailand, Vietnamese told Christians about the role of ancestors in their lives. The Christians brought the Vietnamese to faith by pointing them to God, their greatest ancestor.

The Bible hints at the tendency of the Hebrews to seek guidance from their ancestors. Saul called upon the ancestors via the witch of Endor, and the woman at the well in John 4 reminded Jesus that her ancestors drank at that well.

The Hebrew prophets did not denigrate ancestors or the practice of esteeming them. Instead, they used the ancestors to point to the God who was before everyone. The prophets pointed beyond the leadership of Abraham, Isaac and Jacob when they reminded the Hebrews that the God of Abraham, Isaac and Jacob leads them.

In modern cultures, people also rely on ancestors for inspiration, but in a different way. They do not see ancestors as the living dead, but as symbolically immortal. Martin Luther, John Calvin and John Wesley are symbolically present in developments in Protestant Christian traditions. George Washington, Thomas Jefferson and Abraham Lincoln are symbolically immortal influences in American politics, and Sigmund Freud continues to influence Western psychology. The history of our literature, art and music is filled with people who live through their contributions to our culture.

If we view history in modern cultures redemptively, we must consider God's influence on these people. In doing so, we can remind ourselves that people do not create anything, but rearrange what the Creator has already given us. Management questions then become: What do our rearrangements of the creation say about our relationship with the Creator? Do they affirm or alienate faith? Do they reveal truth? Are they redemptive? Do they point to the Creator who reconciles all things to himself?

Genealogies

Genealogies are another element that influence the environment in which we manage holistic Christian development. Genealogies, like ancestors, are influential in every culture. In primal cultures, their function is similar to that of ancestors, except they are more personalized. They are like addresses: they show where people reside in the culture. The tribe is the city, a clan is the neighborhood and the nuclear family is the street. The person's place within the family is the number.

When the influence of genealogies confronts Western Christians from modern cultures, they often see social hierarchies that perpetuate injustices, which in turn prevent development. In most cultures, genealogies dictate who people associate with, the types of work people do, and their standards of living. Spiritual power also frequently flows through genealogies.

But like addresses everywhere, some genealogies are more prestigious than others. When two people from a primal culture meet, they share their genealogies to understand where each came from, just as people from other cultures tell where they live. They look for possible connections with each other and identify common acquaintances, establishing relationships to define their transactions.

Genealogical influences are historical and universal. Both Matthew and Luke gave addresses for Jesus in their Gospels. Evidently their readers wanted to know whether Jesus had the correct address to be the Messiah. In Islamic cultures, people gain prestige by tracing their genealogy from Mohammed or the Caliphs. Christians identify with the spiritual genealogy of Abraham.

When Kevin Hovey was a missionary in Papua New Guinea, he searched for a credible way to communicate the truth of the gospel. When someone mentioned the importance the people attached to genealogies, Hovey taught the genealogy of Jesus from Luke 3. This impressed the Papua New Guineans. They believed "the genealogies prove that the Bible is true."[7] "Just the fact of such a long and well ordered genealogy as the Luke 3 account," wrote Hovey, "indicates to Papua New Guineans that Jesus was no ordinary man."[8]

Genealogies are spiritually neutral, but are subject to abuse just as other cultural factors are. The task of holistic Christian development, considering this abuse, is to address them with justice.

When I lived in an Islamic culture and needed someone to clean a cesspool, my staff told me a person from a low tribe would do the job. My sense of egalitarianism caused me to feel some contempt for a culture that would relegate its dirty tasks to people who were born with a particular set of genes.

I found I needed to manage my contempt. Cesspool workers live in the less prestigious neighborhoods of any culture. If the system were unjust, we could probably blame the economic system's priorities and values instead of the genealogical structure. The relevant question asks why economic systems reward power and influence instead of labor (I address this problem in chapter seven).

Values

Occupying the middle ground between culture and religion, values are like the spokes between the hub and rim of a wheel—they govern the integrity of cultures and hold them together. When values get lost, cultures—like a wheel—warp.

Many development theorists agree that values are crucial to development; other development theorists believe that development cannot be experienced without a transformation of values.

David C. Korten writes that values are the strategic edge of religiously oriented NGOs (Non-Government Organizations), the agents of holistic Christian development. His conviction complements the views of many Christian development practitioners who cite values as the distinction between Christian and non-Christian development.

Korten claims that values have been neglected because we view development primarily as a financial and technical task. This neglect, he claims, contributes to many current global crises, "in particular a high incidence of communal violence, the destructive use of natural resources, drug abuse, and social injustice."[9] He encourages religiously oriented NGOs that see their roles as "instruments of charity engaged in transferring material resources to those in need"[10] to ask "basic questions about the larger role of religion in dealing with issues of social justice and conflict that are substantial contributors to the conditions of human suffering that most NGOs seek to relieve."[11]

The problem Christians face is naming the values we want to communicate in our work, and inculcating those values in the cultures we are affecting. Christian development, many practitioners claim, focuses on the values of working with integrity, caring for the poorest of the poor, advocating justice, and giving everyone the opportunity to hear the gospel. If we summed up these values in a word, that word is *shalom*— the term that represents or symbolizes the values of our faith.

The effective use of values in managing holistic Christian development is dependent on how we communicate them to people in host cultures. If we show values as the connections between God and our work, are we communicating this relationship in a way that enables the people to see the connections? Are the connections relevant for the situations of the people in the host culture? If the people do not see the values we are communicating, or they perceive the values as irrelevant to their culture, are we miscommunicating our intentions? Are we speaking a language the people do not understand?

When I asked a random sample of Muslims why they thought a Christian development organization was working in their village, they based their answers on their interpretation of the values they saw Christians expressing. Some Muslims saw Christians valuing international relationships. Others thought Christians were earning salvation. A few thought money was the prime value, and a handful saw Christians expressing the need to share their faith through their work.

In another Islamic culture, Western Christians choose to communicate their faith by living at the economic level of the poorest people in the community. They live in simple homes without the comforts of electricity, water or household help.

From a Western cultural perspective, these Christians communicate the values of austerity and asceticism, values that are part of Western spiritual traditions. The impact of this strategy on the Islamic culture depends on how the community sees these values. Does the spiritual history of their culture, like that of Western culture, have traditions that connect asceticism or austerity with spirituality?

When I taught in an Islamic culture, one of my students asked me why my family lived so poorly. We did not think we lived so poorly, but the student believed people who held particular religious or professional positions should have prestigious lifestyles. Our lifestyle was inconsistent with his values. I told the student we lived sacrificially because God provided for our comfort, and we could give the money we did not use on ourselves to other people.

The answer exposed him to another set of values that might have confused him, offended him, or challenged him to transform his values. Its initial effect depended on whether he saw us experiencing God's blessings without the comforts of our modern culture. The second factor was whether our values could point him to a new perspective of God's blessings. Could it transform his idea that spiritual people should have more material comforts than other people?

An example of holistic Christian management

Managing holistic Christian development by transforming values, perceptions of ancestors, and views of genealogies and spirits involves finding elements from the past that give hope for the future. It is analogous to enabling people who view the world from the back of the truck to look forward without losing sight of the past. Conversely, it calls people who drive the truck to sit in the back without losing perspective on the future.

When the Hebrew prophets saw their community was in danger of venerating or worshipping Abraham, Isaac and Jacob, they did not actively discourage people from focusing on the three patriarchs. Instead, they called the people to worship the God of the patriarchs. In this regard, the past pointed toward the future. The God of Abraham, Isaac and Jacob promised the coming of the Messiah.

The New Testament also reflects a future hope from a view of the past. When the disciples were anticipating the loss of Christ, they received the promise of the Holy Spirit. When the early church focused on the past, the Christians received the promise of the second coming of Christ. Throughout Scripture, a focus on the past brings hope for the future.

Holistic Christian development complements Scripture by transforming the glory of the past—or the past's oppressive images—to a future hope. In this regard, holistic Christian development empowers people to see God going before them. It also affirms their hope for the future as they see God in the future, as well as in the past and present.

In a culture similar to the one where I met Sarah, the woman with the *jinn*, the Christian manager of a well-drilling project saw the villagers victimized by their passive acceptance of an environment that was turning into a desert. The land was losing its ability to support the people whose lives depended on it, but the people were helpless to resist what they believed was the will of God.

The problem was understanding God's will instead of the symptoms—the deteriorating environment. In approaching the problem, the manager chose to communicate God's affirmation of the well-drilling project by creating a covenant with the people. This covenant recognized that God was leading the agency and the people to come together as stewards of his creation. Together, in the will of God, they planned their work and organized their resources to work to control the degenerating environment.

The covenant transformed the people's passive view of their oppressive environment by pointing to the God who created the ancestors in an environment that was fruitful. It enabled people to see their spirituality and decisions regarding the well-drilling project not as either-or but as both-and. God controls the environment and gives them responsibility for maintaining it.

With the digging of each well, the community had the opportunity to evaluate their view of God's place in other areas of life. They no longer saw themselves as victims of capricious spirits. The community believed that a curse was on this village. Through the power of God, the agency confronted the curse by drilling a well in that village.

To a significant extent, the well-drilling project enabled the people to transform their view of themselves, their history and the way they understood God's redemptive work in creation. They were not fatalistic in the sense that they saw themselves as victims of external spirits. Instead, they saw themselves participating in the redemptive work of God.

NOTES

1. These diagrams are based on illustrations found in *Phenomenology and Institutions of Folk Religions*, Paul G. Hiebert (Pasadena: Fuller Theological Seminary, 1990), pp. 16 and 22.

2. *Jinn* is an Arabic word for spirit. Spirits are generally perceived to be the counterparts of demons but, unlike demons, *jinn* can be good or bad.

3. John Mbiti believed Africans traditionally had little interest in the future, and whenever Africans today show an interest in the future, it is due to Christianity and Western education (see Benezet Buju, *African Theology in its Social Context* (Maryknoll: Orbis Books, 1992), p. 28).

4. Wade Davis, MD, "The Power to Heal," *Newsweek* (September 24, 1990): 39-40.

5. Ibid.

6. Kivuto Ndeti, "African Traditional Medicine in Modern Medical Training and Practice," *Medical Anthropology*, Francis X. Grollig, S.J., and Francis B. Haley, eds. (The Hague: Mouton Publishers, 1976), pp. 11-26.

7. Kevin G. Hovey, *Before All Else Fails . . . Read the Directions*, (Brisbane: Harvest Publications, 1986), p. 157.

8. Ibid., p. 158.

9. David C. Korten, *Getting to the 21st Century: Voluntary Action and the Global Agenda* (West Hartford: Kumarian Press, 1990), p. 223.

10. Ibid.

11. Ibid.

FIVE

Education:
Liberating and empowering people

"Heaven and earth will pass away,
but my words will never pass away."
Matthew 24:35

A POSTER from Abingdon Press says:

> Books about religion are also about love, sex, politics, AIDS, war,
> peace, justice, ecology, theology, philosophy, addiction, recovery,
> ethics, race, gender, dissent, technology, old age, New Age, faith,
> heavy metal, mortality, beauty, God, psychology, money, dogma,
> freedom, history, death and . . . *Life!*[1]

However, when teachers teach subjects that fall on the physical
side of the physical-spiritual dichotomy—such as politics, ecology and
technology—people frequently ask if these subjects have spiritual components. People ask this question to determine how the ministry is being
spiritualized. How are these topics sanctified, or made Christian? Is the
material taught with Christian values, or does an evangelistic component
of the ministry complement the development component?

All too often, Christians accept so-called secular education as part
of Christian ministry if it has an evangelistic component. This arrange-
ment fills both blocks of the spiritual-physical dichotomy. As Figure 5.1
on page 88 illustrates, when we apply the physical-spiritual dichotomy to
education we create an artificial distinction and divide the holistic nature
of education. Christian education becomes limited to topics that deal
with spiritual issues, and secular education deals with other areas.

Yet Christian education is not dualistic or dichotomous. Instead, it
seeks to understand God's redemptive work in all areas of life.

Figure 5.1   The spiritual-physical dichotomy

Spiritual (supernatural, sacred, values, private)	Physical (natural, secular, facts, public)
Theology Religion Ethics Christian Education	Physical Sciences Social Sciences Economics Management Secular Education
(Evangelism)	*(Development)*

Holistic Christian education is a journey

Holistic Christian education, to use a metaphor from Adam Curle, is a journey. The students and teachers travel together; each knows part of the country. Both students and teachers have ideas and experiences that enable them to make contributions to each other.

The task for teachers is to make the journey meaningful by enabling the students to make relationships between what they know and what they are learning. To do otherwise is an educational failure. Holism sees education in the sense of the Latin word *educo*, which means to raise, lead, bring out, nurture and facilitate growth.

Holistic Christian education further assumes that God reveals truth through his revealed Word and his creation. The journey is through the Bible and through the environments in which we live. The journey starts with indigenous thought patterns and frames of reference, meets the needs of the people, and involves them as active learners.

Holistic education brings *shalom* and empowers people by enabling them to understand how the innovations that others introduce to their culture contribute to their welfare. The basis for holistic education is the belief that all elements of a culture are related. There should be no introduction of an innovation without first understanding how it affects other aspects of the culture.

Recognizing that education addresses a wide range of issues, holistic education, like other aspects of holistic Christian development, answers *why* questions before it answers *how* questions. It tries to learn why particular innovations are important to the cultures that use them, and how these innovations affect the frames of reference within a culture.

People who work in various aspects of development have many stories about development projects taking strange twists. These twists usually cause the projects to fail. Invariably, the failure occurs because project managers pay little attention to how the projects address their beneficiaries' basic assumptions about life. The project beneficiaries usually do not understand the need for the projects. This lack of understanding is often due to development experts designing projects with solutions to problems the people do not believe they have, or that inculcate values the people do not believe they need.

One vivid story is about a reforestation project that planted a few hectares of saplings that survived a major drought. The survival of the trees was a marvelous encouragement to the community leaders who were struggling to protect scarce arable land from further erosion.

Government officials planned a visit to the community to commend the residents for their work. The community prepared to greet the officials in the same manner that the people of Jerusalem greeted Jesus on what has become known as Palm Sunday. The people welcomed their distinguished visitors by waving branches along the roads as the visitors went by. When the officials arrived at the reforestation site, they saw stubs that were once saplings. After the officials left, the villagers used what remained of their reforestation project for firewood.[2]

Undoubtedly, the people in the reforestation project were trained to plant trees, but they were not educated to understand why the trees empowered them and transformed their environment. They never took ownership of the project, but saw it as an item on the agenda of the development agency that implemented it. In this respect, the project was not a liberating force.

Indigenous cultural patterns and frames of reference

Another agency showed a film on health education to a rural African village. The purpose of the film was to encourage people to protect themselves from germs that caused illnesses. The film centered on the transmission of germs from the environment to the human body through insects, dirty water and contaminated food. When the film was over, the health workers solicited the villagers' responses to it. The villagers discussed the sizes and colors of the chickens.

This response stunned the health workers. What did chickens have to do with the film? They reviewed the film, and saw that chickens did appear in a few minor segments.

Why did the villagers focus on the incidentals of the film without grasping its major content? It was because the film made no other reference points to the villagers' culture; chickens were the only item in the film that made sense to them.

People from modern cultures have heard about germs all their lives and some probably have seen germs through a microscope. But what do germs mean to people who have never seen a microscope? The film did not empower people to gain mastery over their environment because it did not recognize the basic assumptions the people made about their environment.

The above examples are characteristic of several failed development projects. The problem is a failure to educate people holistically. Education that is both Christian and holistic enables people to understand how God works redemptively in their culture. The people in the reforestation project, for example, did not see how the trees would contribute to the transformation of their traditions, culture, faith and physical environment.

Criticisms of holistic Christian education

Critics of holistic education argue that the assumptions of this approach to learning lean toward reinventing the wheel. They claim that education does not evolve within a culture, but can be transferred from one culture to another.

These critics substantiate this claim by citing that people do not have to know how to operate a donkey cart before they can drive a car. While this example is true, the proponents of this view are mixing education with training. Of course we can train people to drive a car without their first knowing how to operate a donkey cart, but they have to be educated to understand the integration of cars into their culture. Before they can drive, they must understand something about the organization of their traffic.

We all have stories about traffic situations that confront us in other cultures. We generally tell these stories to illustrate the disorganization of traffic in other cultures. But these stories also illustrate how little we know about the organization of traffic in other cultures. Invariably, the traffic patterns have integrity, but people express this integrity differently throughout various cultures.

One traffic story is told by a Westerner who observed a traffic incident in a major Asian city. It is about the drivers of a motor scooter and a truck confronting each other about the right of way. To the Westerner, the truck driver was on the wrong side of the street, foolishly arguing that he had the right of way. The driver of the scooter seemed to have the more valid argument.

Yet within his culture, the truck driver may have had the right of way. The people of that culture, in contrast to the people of Western cultures, organized traffic by size and speed. Big vehicles have power over little ones; fast ones have power over slow ones. The validity of the truck driver's argument lay in whether the size of his truck had priority over the speed of the scooter.

The conflict between the two drivers had to be worked out within the integrity of their culture. When they finished their argument, both drivers had a new awareness of the traffic rules.[3] But the important point of the story is the role of the person who told it. This person believed he had a solution to the problem that would enlighten both drivers.

Implementing the observer's solution, however, would have deprived the drivers of working out the problem themselves. In the concept of Paulo Freire, they would have suffered from the disempowering effects of "the banking concept of education." The observer, who did not participate in the culture, deposits some knowledge in the minds of those who do participate in the culture. This deprives them of the opportunity to empower themselves by solving their problems.

Holistic Christian education meets the needs of the students

Paulo Freire, author of *Pedagogy of the Oppressed*, wrote this classic book on an approach to education that was both liberating and empowering. This approach liberates people from the shackles of education that are culturally irrelevant. It also empowers them to take control of their learning by gaining and using knowledge to solve the problems they face in their current situations.

In developing this approach to education, Freire contrasted "problem-solving education," which focuses on the needs of the learners, with the "banking concept of education." The banking concept of education leans more toward focusing on the needs of teachers to convey information to their students, regardless of the relevancy of the information. The banking concept of education creates passive learners, while problem-solving education stimulates active learning.

The banking concept of education frustrates holistic Christian education by focusing on what people do not know instead of building on what they do know. It esteems knowledge as "a gift bestowed by those who consider themselves knowledgeable upon those whom they consider to know nothing."[4] More often than not, it meets the needs of the teachers instead of the students. It has a marginalizing, instead of an empowering, effect on people. It breeds contempt instead of *shalom*. It gives the students little opportunity to compare what they learn with the reality of their lives.

The banking concept of education was alive and well in the East African college where I taught. One day, some students wanted to do a marketing research project for a "fast-food" restaurant in a bedroom community (a housing suburb where urban office workers live). The students did not know what fast food was, and could not make a relationship between bedrooms and communities.

"Why do you need to know about bedroom communities?" I asked. "Are we empowering you to live in this culture, or oppressing you by teaching you to solve problems that you do not have?"

An African woman poignantly expressed the oppressive nature of the banking concept of education when she saw the impact her husband's education had on his ability to relate to his family and culture:

> My husband has read much
> He has read extensively and deeply
> He has read among whiteman
> And he is clever like whiteman
> And the reading has killed my man
> In the ways of his people
> He has become a stump . . .
>
> The deadly vengeance ghosts
> of the writers
> Will capture your head
> and like my husband
> You will become a walking corpse
> For all our young men
> Were finished in the forest
> Their manhood was finished
> In the classrooms[5]

Involving students as active learners

Freire writes that we must replace the banking concept of education with *problem-posing education*. "In problem-posing education [people] develop their power to perceive critically the way they exist in the world with which and, in which, they find themselves."[6]

In this approach to education, teachers do not give students a large quantity of information that is not relevant to the students' situations. Instead, teachers guide the students through a process of reflection, action and reflection. The process enables the students to solve the problems they confront. In the banking concept of education, students miss the *why* of their education. In problem-solving education, *why* is a central issue.

Making education holistic by involving students is a challenge for all teachers. Jesus modeled this form of education. He said: "Heaven and earth will pass away, but my words will never pass away" (Matt. 24:35).

This statement is outrageous if we consider that Jesus did not write anything, and those closest to him wrote almost a generation after his death. But his words endured. His example empowered the people who followed him and listened to him, enabling them to make relationships between a broad range of issues that he addressed.

How did Jesus educate his audience to make his words endure? Did his audience take volumes of notes on everything he said?

This is unlikely; most of them were probably illiterate. It is more likely that he educated them according to their thought patterns and situations. He empowered, challenged, confronted and affirmed his audience by using parables, proverbs, prayers, symbols and signs they could grasp. He addressed their needs and actively involved them in his teachings.

He told farmers who struggled with unbelief that their faith needed to be the size of a mustard seed—a concept they readily understood. Merchants who transported their wares on the backs of camels easily envisioned the relationship between the size of camels and the eyes of needles. They got the point of Jesus' message comparing rich people going to heaven and camels fitting through the eyes of needles. It pierced their thoughts about the relationship between their wealth and faith.

Jesus told the Pharisees who scorned the presence of tax collectors and sinners stories about lost coins, lost sheep and lost sons. They saw the graphic connection between Jesus' teachings and their lives. They saw that peace with God called them to be at peace with each other.

Holistic educators actively involve their students in their lessons by finding culturally relevant media. People do not grasp the content of a message unless teachers communicate it through media the people can understand.

Literacy and Christian education

Literacy is central to Christian education because it is an essential tool in empowering people to understand God's redemptive work in creation. Christians often teach literacy to enable people to read the Bible. Yet an important additional value to literacy training is empowering people to understand, value and preserve the oral traditions of their culture.

The preservation of these traditions gives people dignity by affirming how God values them as people. It also affirms that their cultures participate in the redemptive work of God through Christ. Lamin Sanneh focuses on Bible translation and literacy as major contributions of Western missionaries. He wrote:

The importance of the vernacular translation was that . . . local believers acquired new interest, not only in the vernacular [translation], but also in recording their history and collecting accounts of indigenous wisdom . . .

Here is an acute paradox: the vernacular Scriptures and the wider cultural and linguistic enterprise on which translation rested provided the means and occasion for arousing a sense of national pride, yet, it was the missionaries—foreign agents—who were the creators of the entire process . . .

The impact of the translation process is, indeed, incalculable. Suddenly hitherto illiterate populations were equipped with a written Scripture for the first time, and from the wonder and pride of possessing something new that is also strangely familiar, they burst upon the scene with confidence in the who and why of their existence.[7]

The intrinsic power of words

While stories abound about misfortunes that literacy could have prevented, I want to focus on how non-literate people use written words. People who do not have adequate levels of literacy, as the following stories show, have developed a variety of uses for the Bible and other written materials.

Non-literate people often value written material because they believe the words are intrinsically powerful. In Haiti, Christians place the Bible under their pillows to ward off evil spirits and bad dreams while they sleep. One mother said her children's nightmares stopped after she placed an open Bible above the door of the house. There are stories of other mothers who tear a page out of the Bible, boil it in water like a cup of tea, and drink it as medicine.

Even non-Christians want to buy a Bible and have it in their homes because they think it will protect them. They do not read it and will even try to keep people from opening it. Sometimes people are buried with a Bible in their coffin to protect them from evil or punishment.[8] These people understand the Bible has power, but they do not understand why it does. Until they learn how to read, they have little basis to distinguish between the magical power of their religious traditions and the redemptive power of Christ.

Muslims from non-Arabic cultures who do not understand the Arabic language have similar uses for the Qur'an. They frequently memorize major parts of the Qur'an in Arabic without knowing the meanings of the words or verses they are memorizing. They believe the words of the Qur'an have power apart from the meanings. There is no need for the people who are reciting the words of the Qu'ran to understand what the words mean. When properly articulated, these Muslims believe the words and meanings effect change in any given situation.

Mothers bring sick children to have Qur'an verses spoken over them; travellers have verses recited to insure safe journeys, and people sleep over Qur'anic verses to ward off spirits. I once attended a wedding where a sheikh spat into a bowl of water as he recited Qur'anic verses. The couple drank the water at the end of their wedding ceremony, consuming the power of the Qur'an into their marriage.

The idea that words have intrinsic power pervades many areas of life. Muslim leaders who oppose Christianity are willing to have Christians pray blessings on their homes.

In one African country, a government planned to raze a mosque to use the land on which it stood for other purposes. The Islamic community asked Christians to encircle the mosque and pray for it. After the prayers the government chose to use another parcel of land. Were the Muslims impressed by the power of the God to whom the Christians prayed? I don't think so; they were probably more impressed with the words the Christians used.

One of the problems we face in basing education on literacy is the time required to help a significant portion of the world's population become literate. Currently, about 20 percent of the world's population is illiterate; about 98 percent of the world's literate population live in industrialized countries.[9]

This gap between the literate and non-literate populations of the world challenges us to continue our literacy programs, and to find ways of teaching people who are not literate. Meeting this challenge involves educating people through the media they use to communicate with each other.

In many cultures, these media include stories, proverbs and parables that form the basis of their beliefs, values, ideas, knowledge and wisdom. The following section proposes how we can use indigenous myths to communicate God's redemptive plan through holistic Christian education.

On educating the Bozos

The Bozos are an ethnic group of about 100,000 people who live along the Niger River in Mali. For centuries, the Bozos have fished in the local rivers. For the Bozos, fishing is more than an occupation: it is an identity. The stories, myths, parables and proverbs of the Bozos revolve around fish. If a Bozo man cannot fish, he is not sure he can be a Bozo any longer.

The supply of fish in the rivers is currently being depleted. The Bozos have not developed any methods to conserve the natural supply of fish. A dam up the river—which has done wonders for irrigation—has re-duced the flow of water and stopped the normal migrations of what the Bozos believe is the staff of life.

The lack of fish is causing the Bozo culture to disintegrate. The Bozos who are in their most productive years have left the villages for urban centers. Others have become nomadic, searching the rivers throughout the region for better fishing conditions. A few Bozos have resorted to agriculture. The Bozos who remain in the their villages are among the poorest people in the country.

A few development agencies have attempted to educate the Bozos. Most of the education programs started with literacy training. Literacy is a valuable skill for the Bozos, but the development agencies implemented the training in a way that came closer to the banking concept of education than to problem-solving education. Therefore, the Bozos did not see any connection between literacy and fishing, and soon lost interest in literacy training.

If we examine how we can implement literacy as problem-solving education, we should consider how literacy empowers the Bozos to solve their problems as they understand them. The central problem is how literacy increases the supply of fish.

When the Bozos discuss why the fish supply is depleting, they will invariably discuss the dams. They know the dams are stopping the water, which prevents the fish from migrating. But they are powerless to address how the dams affect their culture because their religious traditions prevent them from being innovative, and their illiteracy prevents them from participating in the political arena.

The problem of religious traditions stems from the assumptions the Bozos make about their traditions. The stories in their religious traditions tell how their ancestors gave future generations of Bozos the power to catch fish. These stories are the pulse of Bozo culture. They explain how things came to be, and why things are the way they are. If these stories were written, the Bozos would find literacy much more appealing and useful.

Yet if Christian development practitioners translated these stories, they would raise questions about why Christians should translate non-Christian myths and stories. The initial answer, as previously discussed, is that education must address the problems as the learners see them. But this answer does not stop with this initial solution. The answer also gives the Bozos an opportunity to learn how their ancestors point to God, the Creator of the fish.

This belief that God existed before the Bozos' ancestors is an important aspect of problem-solving education. It gives Christians the opportunity to help the Bozos graft their history into the story of God's redemptive work in creation. The Bozos' stories only go as far as their ancestors. They explain why the Bozos fish, but they do not explain why the fish are diminishing, leaving the Bozos helpless to solve the problems that threaten their existence.

The story that gives the Bozos a basis to work toward solving their problems is the story that tells about the God who created a good creation that fell because of sin. This story puts the lack of fish in the context of a fallen creation that God is reconciling and redeeming through Christ.

The fish that provide the basis for the Bozos' subsistence are essential elements of the creation that God is redeeming through Christ. However, all elements of the Bozo culture are fallen, yet also participate in God's redemptive plan. This redemptive plan provides for the temporal and eternal dimensions of life in the Bozo culture.

The Bozos can implement this redemptive plan in a number of ways. One way is to develop effective methods of conserving fish. Another is by artificially cultivating fish. Finally, the Bozos may see God's redemptive plan empowering them to liberate themselves from their fishing traditions, and participating in agriculture.

The specific method of implementing a redemptive plan for the Bozos, or any other culture, is incidental to their ability to experience *shalom*. The major concern is that people participate in education programs that meet their needs, incorporate their experience and knowledge, and involves them as active learners and problem-solvers. The final step is enabling people to liberate and empower themselves to interpret educational programs as part of the redemptive work of God through Christ.

NOTES

1. Abingdon Press, Nashville, 1990.

2. This story is from a private newsletter by a World Vision staff member in West Africa.

3. The development of this story is based on: Paul G. Hiebert, "Traffic Patterns in Seattle and Hyderabad: Immediate and Mediate Transactions," *Journal of Anthropological Research*, University of New Mexico, Vol. 32:4 (October 1976): 326-336.

4. Paulo Freire, *Pedagogy of the Oppressed* (New York: Herder and Herder, 1970), p. 58.

5. Herbert V. Klem, *Oral Communication of the Scripture* (Pasadena: William Carey Library, 1982), p. 160.

6. Freire, p. 71.

7. Lamin Sanneh, "Christian Missions and the Western Guilt Complex," *The Christian Century* (April 8, 1987): 331-332.

8. *Pulse*, Vol. 26 (February 8, 1991): 3.

9. John Kenyon, "Toward the Light of Literacy," *Together*, Vol. 29 (January-March 1989): 1.

SIX

The environment:
Caring for creation

God saw all that he had made, and it was very good. . . .
Genesis 1:31

". . . Your will be done on earth as it is in heaven."
Matthew 6:10

For the creation was subjected to frustration,
not by its own choice,
but by the will of the one who subjected it,
in hope that the creation itself
will be liberated from its bondage to decay
and brought into the glorious freedom of the children of God.
Romans 8:20-21

The nations were angry; and your wrath has come.
The time has come for judging . . .
and for destroying those who destroy the earth.
Revelation 11:18

". . . CREATION ITSELF will be liberated from its bondage to decay and brought into the glorious freedom of the children of God" (Rom. 8:21). This verse came to mind when I participated in a famine relief effort in East Africa. I visited a group of nomadic families who had gathered around some wells to receive assistance from a food distribution project. All creation, I realized, participates in the redemptive work of God.

The above verse from Romans 8 brought hope to a situation that seemed hopeless. The malnutrition among the people was severe. The children were more seriously affected than the adults. The few animals that managed to survive were emaciated; many died.

"Does God care about the physical welfare of these people?" I wondered. "What about the environment they live in? We cannot separate the people from their environment, and this environment is causing them to perish."

After I spent a night guarding a herd of camels with the men, we made a pitifully desperate attempt to milk the beasts. Camels have a reputation for supplying all the food that is necessary for the human diet. After squeezing a few drops of the precious liquid into a bowl, the men told me that the camels had not eaten well enough to produce much milk.

That was an understatement. I scanned the landscape, and saw trees and bushes stripped of their leaves, buds and bark. The range had turned to dust.

One of the men reminisced about the days when the community prospered. He told me a story about a tree that perpetually grew leaves. When the camels ate the leaves, the milk was always sweet. That tree had died long ago.

"Now," I thought, "is the time to find such a tree."

The sentiments of the community did not reflect *shalom*. The government's emphasis on settlement and agriculture squeezed the nomads onto smaller portions of the poorest land. They saw themselves as fighting an environment that could no longer support them; they had little hope for improved conditions.

"Is there grazing in the foothills?" I asked a group of men who were tending the camels.

"The camels and goats cannot get there," replied a spokesperson for the group, reflecting the people's attitude of having been defeated by a hostile environment.

"Why not?"

"Forty percent of our herds have died; the animals are weak and their hooves will wear out if they move."

"How many camels and goats did you have?"

"Eighty camels and two hundred goats," they replied.

"Are you slaughtering the animals before they die?" I asked.

"People who eat weak animals will become weak themselves," came the impatient retort.

"What are you eating?"

"Our tongues have not tasted food for several days."

"How can I help you?" I asked.

Raising his forefinger toward the sky, the spokesperson said, "You cannot help us—we depend only on God."

Perhaps he was right. He was among the millions of people

throughout the world who will suffer or die because of environmental degradation. International assistance could provide this man and his community with enough food to survive until the next rains came, but the people were suffering from the environmental decay that results from overpopulated, overgrazed and deforested land. Food distribution, as important as it was, was only a temporary solution. It was tantamount to providing a band-aid for a hemorrhage.

The environment is of vital concern to Christian holism

Christian development cannot be holistic without a concern for the environment. Holism (Figure 6.1), in contrast to the dualistic world view of the Western world (Figure 6.2), is a model that meets this concern. In holism, all the elements of creation participate in the redemptive plan of God. The physical elements of creation do not receive salvation in the sense that God resurrects them to eternal life. Instead, holism supports the belief that all the elements of creation—the seen and the unseen—participate in God's redemptive work through Christ.

Dualism, the model that has characterized the Christian response to the environment, is simply inadequate to communicate the fullness of God's redemptive plan for creation. Dualism limits redemption to the

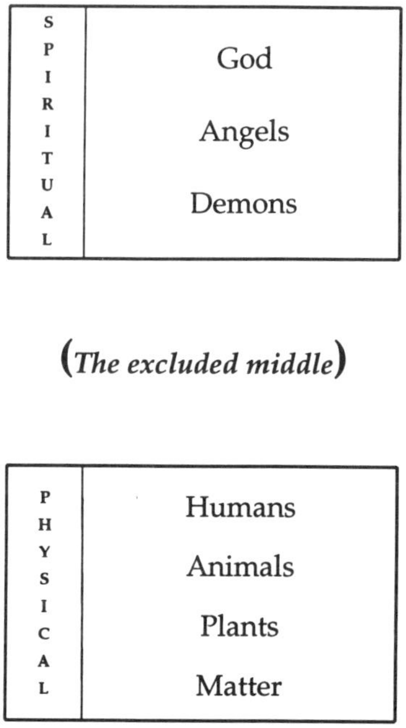

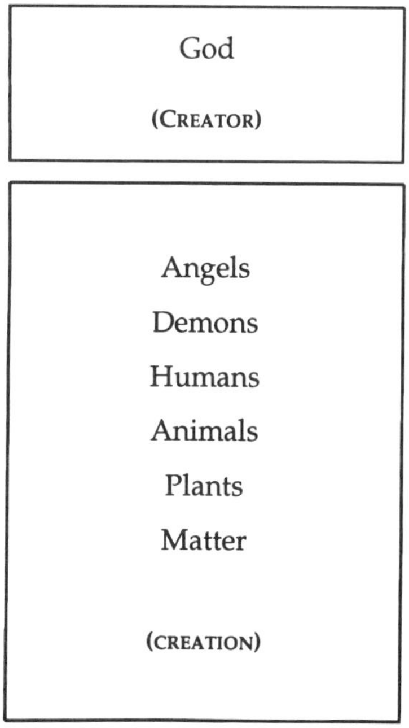

Figure 6.1   Holistic world view   Figure 6.2   Dualistic world view

spiritual dimension of creation, the top box (see Figure 6.2). Under dualism, when God redeems people they move through some sense of spiritual rebirth from the bottom box to the top box, leaving the bottom box out of God's redemptive plan.

Dualism gives little or no thought to restoring the physical elements of creation to the purpose for which God created them. In a dualistic universe, creation becomes like a building that is burning out of control—the people must be rescued before they are destroyed with the building. Holism, in extending God's redemptive plan to every aspect of creation, recognizes the integrated and interdependent nature of the elements of creation.

The interdependent nature of the eco-crisis

While environmental issues are essential to holistic Christian development, environmental components cannot simply be tacked onto development projects. We must integrate them into the many issues that address holistic Christian development's concern for sustaining life. The environment, and the people who depend on it—all of us—do not live in isolation from the other issues of holistic Christian development. Just as hunger problems are not only agricultural, environmental problems are not only ecological. Environmental problems are theological, political, economic and cultural.

We have to balance the ecological and environmental aspects of holistic Christian development with other aspects. One aspect cannot take priority over the other, but each has to represent the long-term and short-term interests of the people who are participating in the projects. We must address ecological problems in view of the short-term, and more immediate, needs of the people. When a leader of a group of rural workers from Brazil met a group of North American ecologists, he said: "These ecologists from the United States and Europe do not care about the people of Brazil . . . We have to survive—to survive now."[1]

A recent issue of *Africa Report* expressed similar sentiments. The author cited a survey from the United Nations Environment Programme that revealed "only in Africa were people not willing to make material sacrifices for the sake of the environment. The standard of living in Africa today has declined compared to 10 years ago or even 20 years ago."[2] The people are less willing to make short-term sacrifices, despite expected long-term gains.

A proverb attributed to several sources says: "We do not inherit the land from our ancestors; we borrow it from our children." The children of every culture are likely to inherit land that is progressively losing its ability to support life. We have all read statistics about the amount of soil we lose to erosion, the scarcity of clean water, and the tons of pollution we dump into the air we breathe. The recent edition of *State of the World* included some alarming statistics:

> During the 20 years since the first Earth Day, in (April) 1970, the world lost nearly 200 million hectares of tree cover . . . Deserts expanded by some 120 million hectares, claiming more land than is currently planted in crops in China. Thousands of plant and animal species with which we shared the planet in 1970 no longer exist . . . And the world's farmers lost an estimated 480 billion tons of topsoil, roughly equivalent to the amount of India's cropland.[3]

Ulrich Duchrow and Gerhard Liedke wrote:

> Today's destruction of the environment differs from all earlier destruction of the environment because it is systematic, faster than the natural regulating mechanism, and is of worldwide dimensions. The ozone layer is still seriously endangered. The consequences of acid rain are worsening. Over-fishing in many waters is increasingly the rule. Pollution of coastal waters is increasing.[4]

As convincing as they are, statistics have a way of masking reality. They attach desensitizing numbers to conditions that affect our lives in a serious way.

Understanding the eco-crisis

Let's change our approach to understanding the eco-crisis, and look at some metaphors that will communicate the gravity of the current state of the environment.

Some people have said that the planet is like a sinking ship. This metaphor is good, but it is inadequate. It affirms the idea that somehow creation is incidental to our survival and salvation. It fails to communicate how we depend on the earth for our survival, and how God's redemptive work in creation regenerates both the earth and humankind. The sinking ship metaphor leads us to believe that "we can be independent from nature," that we "can improve upon nature's systems," and that we "can get more out of a system than we put into it."[5]

Most of us who find ourselves on a sinking ship care more about being rescued than we care about the ship itself. We approach the crisis economically. We insure our interests to minimize our losses. Our concerns are the adequacy of lifeboats, the availability of helicopters and whether we can salvage our belongings. After the rescue effort, our lives go on. In the eco-crisis, the earth is not an incidental vessel. There are no lifeboats, and there's no safe haven. We cannot approach the eco-crisis economically; our interests cannot be insured, nor our losses minimized.

We need another metaphor to describe the crisis in the environment, a metaphor that focuses on stewardship.

Think of the earth as a spaceship.[6] Spaceships, like the earth, travel through the galaxy without lifeboats. They are not incidental vessels; they are vital to the well-being and survival of their passengers, and there is no rescue from them when they disintegrate.

We value spaceships the way we should value the earth. A spaceship, like the earth, is an integrated network of individual parts that contribute to the functioning of the entire unit. Each part is important, and we value each for its own merit, and for its contribution to the whole. We recognize that spaceships give us no more than what we put into them, and we affirm that our survival depends on the integrity of its makers. Our view of the earth is also a reflection of our belief in the integrity of the One who created it.

Environmental problems are theological

Perhaps no issue has suffered more from a dualistic world view than the environmental issue. A study cited by Wesley Granberg-Michaelson in *Tending the Garden* showed that people who attend church—North Americans, I assume—have a lower view of non-human life and the environment than those who do not attend church. Granberg-Michaelson uses this study to imply that most people have simply dropped a view of creation from the theological equation.

The absence of a theological view of creation leaves Christians with a variety of ideas about the environment. The dualistic influence of ancient Greece continues to prevail among modern Christians. In this view, the earth, disconnected from spiritual redemption, becomes an object that God created primarily for humanity to exploit. Only the "spiritual" is worth saving, and matter contributes nothing essential to the process of salvation.[7]

Yet matter does contribute to our salvation. The actual body of Christ was physical, and rose physically. We cannot maintain a high view of the incarnation while having a low view of creation. This incongruency leads us to an abstract, intellectual orthodoxy that "seems to suggest that God really did not need to come and live with us. We dare not belittle the power of the verbal message, but if this can carry the freight along, then God went to a lot of needless humiliation and suffering."[8]

Putting the environment back into the theological equation calls for us to change our language, and to get a biblical perspective on creation. The central problem is understanding the effect of the Fall on creation. Not many of us discount that the Fall affected creation, but we are less prone to seeing how creation also participates in redemption.

The biblical view of creation is analogous to that of a child who gets a degenerative illness after she is born.[9] The child's appearance changes over time, but the relationship between child and parents remains one of unconditional love and enduring commitment. The parents care for the child, love the child as she is, and never give up hope that the child will have a fulfilling life. If the child is cured, the parents rejoice.

God saw creation as good (Gen. 1:31). It is his handiwork; it is not autonomous from him or antagonistic to his purposes. Instead, he created it by the power of his word from chaos to order, for his will to be fulfilled.

God intended creation to be fertile; the creatures that inhabited the earth were to be fruitful and multiply. Humankind would have dominion over creation to insure the fulfillment of this purpose. This dominion implies a sense of stewardship and dependence. Creation is not subject to the whims of humankind, but we are responsible for using it to fulfill the will of God. We are to see that we do not lose creation's fertility because of our irresponsible stewardship.

After the Fall, creation became subject to decay and disintegration. But like parents who stay committed to a sick child, God's commitment to creation continues. He sustains it, and it reflects his glory.

God did not abandon creation. Creation participates in the redemption that God provided through Christ. The "victory over sin and death, won on the cross, and seen in the resurrection, must eventually involve nothing less than the transformation of the created order. For this consummation, the creation awaits with eager longing."[10]

Environmental problems are cultural

A primary cause of the eco-crisis is the resistance of people to the idea of altering their lives to insure the survival of the planet. We have an idea—perhaps a fantasy—that the environment can absorb any abuse we give it.

We must check the notion that the earth can absorb unlimited abuse against the harmful effects of unmanaged growth. The concept of unmanaged growth is based on the cultural value that all growth is good. Yet like everything else, we must value growth for its contributions to the holistic nature of human life.

In developed societies, we achieve the fantasy of equating growth with goodness when we consider that agricultural production has grown if yields rise. While higher yields can be good, they depend on a limited creation. Therefore, natural resources have to be transformed to produce growth. The use of natural resources might not be worth the benefits of growth. Agricultural growth, for example, causes soil depletion and erosion. If we weighed the costs of depleting soil against the benefits of higher agricultural yields, we may not consider growth to be such a good thing.

We must evaluate the value of commercial and industrial growth in a way that is similar to agricultural growth—weighing the cost of growth against its consequences.

For example, we consider growth in medical services to be a good thing. But we equally value the industrial and commercial growth that causes health problems and the growth of the medical services that we use to cure those health problems. We place an equal value on the growth in the causes of a problem and the growth in the cures of a problem.

Perhaps modern societies should take the step of evaluating growth according to the costs of achieving it. This step would challenge us to realize that growth has environmental costs. While natural resources are available for people to exploit, they are not cost-free. We use them at the cost of their present and future benefits.

"It is hard to visualize that a meal in one's favorite fast food restaurant damages the tropical forest."[11] Yet throughout the world, 42 percent[12] of the tropical rain forests have been razed for agricultural purposes, primarily to produce inexpensive beef. If we could attach a value to the rain forests that are destroyed to produce this beef, we would get a more accurate measurement of the beef's cost. The beef would be expensive, and we would discourage its increased production.

In primal cultures, this idea that growth is good manifests itself in perpetuating traditions that are detrimental to the environment.

The nomads mentioned at the beginning of the chapter valued the growth of their herds beyond the ability of the environment to support the animals. Camels were the sustenance and pride of their lives. While the animals provided milk, food and leather products, they were also a measure of a family's social status and wealth. Camels are a dignified dowry for any bride and a stable medium of exchange in an inflationary economy. The nomads saw more as simply better. But having more camels was detrimental to the environment.

According to this culture's values, people had social esteem according to the number of animals they owned. These values had to be modified according to the number of animals the environment could sustain. The problem was in defining the ideal number of livestock the environment could sustain instead of attempting to maintain a maximum number for the family and clan's social status.

By expecting that they could maintain a herd of 200 goats and 80 camels, the nomads I visited continued a tradition the environment could no longer support. For centuries, these nomads crossed the land with their camels and goats, constantly moving to allow the land to regenerate. Dry spells created a natural culling of the herds, reducing their sizes to numbers the land could sustain. Rain enabled the environment to support larger herds.

The environment's natural management of the herds would continue—it could not be pushed beyond its limits. The nomads, therefore, had to accept the environment's new rules. They could not continue to fight against an environment that could not support them or their cultural practices. Instead, they had to make peace with the environment by seeing their cultural practices as negotiable items, submitting to the environment's present abilities, and allowing the environment to regenerate.

Environmental problems are economic

Solving environmental problems is like solving hunger problems. People often wonder why humankind can send people to the moon, but we cannot feed the hungry people in the world.

The answer is a matter of economics. We have an economy that supports a trip to the moon, but we are still searching for a politically and economically viable way to eliminate hunger. In the modern world, if a solution to a hunger problem, an environmental problem, or any other type of problem is not economic, we do not consider it a viable option. E. F. Schumacher eloquently illustrated this point by writing:

> It is hardly an exaggeration to say that, with increasing affluence, economics has moved into the very centre of public concern, and economic performance, economic growth, economic expansion, and so forth have become the abiding interest, if not the obsession, of all modern societies. In the current vocabulary of condemnation there are few words as final and conclusive as the word "uneconomic." If an activity has been branded as uneconomic, its right to existence is not merely questioned but energetically denied. Anything that is found to be an impediment to economic growth is a shameful thing, and if people cling to it, they are thought of as either saboteurs or fools. Call a thing immoral or ugly, soul-destroying or a degradation of man, a peril to the peace of the world or to the well-being of future generations; as long as you have not shown it to be "uneconomic" you have not really questioned its right to exist, grow and prosper.[13]

While Schumacher was undoubtedly correct, his position in life enabled him to take advantage of a privilege few people have. His economic resources enabled him to make decisions that reflected values that were either uneconomic or non-economic. Decisions that caused him to spend more money or other resources for purposes that assisted the greater good did not threaten his welfare.

But for the people that holistic Christian development serves, the option of being uneconomic is not so readily available. They have to sacrifice long-term environmental benefits for short-term economic benefits. They have to balance the opportunity costs[14] of being environmentally sound against the opportunity costs of being uneconomic. This tension creates a constant struggle between their values and the reality of their situations.

The opportunity costs of environmentally sound development are high. These costs force people to make choices they would rather not make. If a peasant woman must choose between chopping down a tree or paying a day's wage for another type of fuel, she has a high opportunity cost despite the choice she makes. She would prefer to use another type of fuel. In the long-term, she will benefit from this choice. But in the short term, chopping down the tree looks appealing. She cannot afford to spend a day's wage on fuel.

In a refugee project, a development agency traded the opportunity to purchase medical supplies for the opportunity to buy solar panels. They installed the panels to provide energy in strategic places in the camp. In the long term, it was an environmentally sound decision. In the short term, however, it took money away from other vital services, such as medical care. The incongruity of having solar energy at the expense of having medical supplies and equipment caused dissatisfaction among both the refugees and many development practitioners.

Implementing environmentally sound development

Being stewards of God's creation compels practitioners of holistic Christian development to be environmentally sensitive. At least, the projects should do no environmental damage. At most, the projects should regenerate a decaying environment as much as possible.

Practitioners of holistic Christian development can have environmentally sensitive projects that are also economically, culturally and politically sensitive. The World Vision Oasis project in Menaka, Mali, is a prime example. Drought, desertification, population increases and other environmental stresses have caused the people's environment, and their nomadic way of life, to collapse. The environment could not continue to support the people or their herds.

The Menaka Oasis project responded to regenerating the environment by focusing on range management, livestock breeding, reforestation, water resource development, soil and energy conservation, and agriculture. Building domed houses out of clay, an abundant resource in the environment, was the most innovative aspect of this project. The structures are completely free of wood, a resource that was critically scarce.

In a refugee camp in Africa occupied by former nomads, a forestry project was successful because it addressed the relationship between spirituality, culture, the economic needs of the people, and the need to restore the environment. The refugees were folk Muslims who distrusted Christians, particularly Christians who encouraged them to plan for the future, settle the land, or plant trees. For the past several centuries, the nomads and their ancestors crossed the land with their camels, sheep and goats, constantly moving to allow the land to regenerate. Though it was never abundantly productive, the nomads never taxed the land beyond its capacity to bear witness to Allah's provision.

Christian project personnel proposed the idea of planting trees in the camp to benefit the present and future generations. The nomads understood this proposal to suggest that they should take responsibility for their future. In their minds, this suggestion implied that Allah's provisions were inadequate. Settling the land, planting trees and planning their future was meddling in Allah's affairs. Only his will influenced the next minute of life. In response to the suggestion, one woman said: "How can I see into the future? Only Allah and the government can control what will happen to me. I cannot do anything to change my life."

The project personnel addressed the concerns of this woman, and others like her, by affirming that Allah's provisions were adequate in every respect. Yet the personnel added two challenges that gave the people a new perspective on their faith.

The first challenge was suggesting that the God of the Christians and Muslims had faith in them, and gave them the responsibility of planning their future. This suggestion made enough sense to the people to motivate them to listen further. They always believed they had faith in Allah, but the idea that Allah had faith in them was new. This idea opened them to the biblical teaching that God had given people dominion over the earth, trusting them to care for the environment.

With a twist on their view of faith, the project personnel enabled the refugees to transform their belief that only Allah could plant trees and care for the environment. The refugees believed that God had given them permission, and had the expectation that they would take responsibility to care for his creation.

The second challenge was suggesting that the refugees should trust Allah to provide for them, not only for a season, but for the coming years and decades. This suggestion stemmed from the idea that people planted vegetables and trusted Allah to provide rain for a season. Yet they were not ready to stretch their view of Allah's provision by making a long-term commitment to plant trees for their future, and for the future of their children and grandchildren. The people responded to this challenge, and cooperated in the tree-planting efforts.

In accepting the challenge to take responsibility for their part of the environment, the nomads depended on the sovereign God who gave them dominion over creation. In doing so, they transformed their land, and their faith. They experienced a greater realization of *shalom*, not simply by understanding that God gives peace in a spiritual sense, but also that peace comes through living in an environment that God is restoring to fulfill the purpose for which he created it.

NOTES

1. "Ecologists and the Rain Forest," *Christian Century* (November 6, 1991): 1020.

2. Nomsa Daniels, "Guardians of Eden," *Africa Report* (September-October 1991): 17.

3. Lester R. Brown, ed., *State of the World* (New York: Norton and Company, 1991), p. 3.

4. Ulrich Duchrow and Gerhard Liedke, *Shalom: Biblical Perspectives on Creation, Justice and Peace* (Geneva: WCC Publications, 1987), pp. 16-17.

5. Art and Jocele Meyer, *Earthkeepers: Environmental Perspectives on Hunger, Poverty and Injustice* (Scottdale: Herald Press, 1991), p. 11.

6. The spaceship analogy is by Kenneth Boulding. It is quoted by David Korten in *Getting to the 21st Century: Voluntary Action and the Global Agenda* (West Hartford: Kumarian Press, 1990), p. 33.

7. Philip N. Joranson and Ken Butigan, *The Cry of the Environment: Rebuilding the Christian Creation Tradition* (Santa Fe: Bear Publications, 1984), p. 117.

8. James E. Metzler, *From Saigon to Shalom* (Scottdale: Herald Press, 1985), p. 119.

9. The child analogy is from Albert M. Wolters, *Creation Regained* (Grand Rapids: Wm. B. Eerdmans Co., 1985).

10. William A. Dyrness, *Let the Earth Rejoice: A Biblical Theology of Holistic Mission* (Westchester: Crossway Books, 1983), p. 43.

11. Sean McDonagh, *To Care for the Earth: A Call to a New Theology* (London: Geoffrey Chapman, 1986), p. 35.

12. This figure is from Duchrow and Liedke, p. 16.

13. E.F. Schumacher, *Small is Beautiful: Economics as if People Mattered* (New York: Harper and Row, 1973), p. 39-40.

14. An opportunity cost is defined as the cost of doing one thing rather than

another. If a person gives up a job to become a missionary, the difference between the salary from the job the person gave up and mission support is the cost of accepting the opportunity to be a missionary. When people choose to modify their lives for the sake of the environment, the cost of modifying their lives—whether monetary or otherwise—is an opportunity cost.

SEVEN

Economics:
Making the worldly philosophy holy

. . . Seek justice, encourage the oppressed.
Defend the cause of the fatherless,
plead the case of the widow.
Isaiah 1:17

Now this was the sin of your sister Sodom:
She and her daughters were arrogant,
overfed and unconcerned;
they did not help the poor and needy.
Ezekiel 16:49

"Sir," the invalid replied,
"I have no one to help me into the pool . . .
. . . someone else goes down ahead of me."
John 5:7

LIKE THE MAN who sat powerlessly at the edge of the pool waiting for someone to help him into it, people throughout the world are powerless to improve the quality of their lives. They have little power to compete in an economic system that increasingly disempowers them, and they have no one to help them. How do we communicate the good news of a gospel that makes a covenant of peace by harmonizing creation to such people?

A mother with several children sells a few yards of cloth at the market. She used to make a meager living by buying the cloth at one price and selling it for another. But the demand for clothing in her village is dwindling. Several people who have purchased sewing machines are making clothing that competes with her prices. Some merchants are also importing clothing. The woman's former customers are buying complete garments for a little more than the price of her unimproved cloth.

The woman has the potential to be a skilled seamstress and would like to make dresses. The money she needs to buy a sewing machine, however, is equal to her annual income. What can she do?

A visiting evangelist proclaimed that ". . . my God will meet all your needs according to his glorious riches in Christ Jesus" (Phil. 4:19). It was a great promise, but the evangelist left before she could get a sewing machine. Was his message good news to her? "Can God provide me with a sewing machine?" she wondered. "Does he care if I have an income? Or is the promise to meet our needs limited to what the evangelist called 'spiritual needs?' Does the God whom the evangelist proclaimed make exceptions and provide for material needs?"

Does God limit his concern to spiritual or physical needs?

The questions the woman pondered raise the issue of whether God limits his commitment to spiritual needs, or whether physical needs are also his concern. Undoubtedly, the evangelist would agree that all her needs are God's concern, but he is likely to call physical needs her "felt needs." Felt needs are those that she perceives, and ones that should be met simply because she can perceive her spiritual needs after her felt, physical needs are met.

The problem with this approach is that it cannot acknowledge the validity of her physical needs in the context of *shalom*. Instead, it creates a dichotomy between physical and spiritual—or felt and actual—needs, and uses the meeting of physical needs as a way to meet spiritual needs. It makes development a road to evangelism, instead of acknowledging that the woman's physical and spiritual needs cannot be separated.

This approach does not acknowledge how bringing a sense of well-being to the woman is an essential part of Christian mission. The sewing machine that brings peace to her is not incidental to making God known to her. It is the primary means through which she realizes how God will meet her needs.

People in a West African village, like many throughout the world, do not make distinctions between physical and spiritual needs. The unseen, spiritual world dictates the seen, physical world. In this particular village, huge amounts of rice were rotting because people were not eating or selling it.

A visiting economist asked why the people were not selling the rice. The villagers evaded the question; either no one had an answer for it, or no one wanted to offer one. The visitor, not realizing the message of silence was as powerful as a spoken message, told the village leaders about the economic concept of comparative advantage.[1] He said the village would benefit by selling rice to other villages.

The village leaders nodded, giving the visitor the impression they understood a concept of modern economics. After the village leaders learned a few basic economic principles, the visitor thought, they could develop a strategy to export their rice to other regions.

But the response of the village leaders was less than enthusiastic. Upon further discussion, the visitor learned that the people believed the spirits who had the power to make rice grow also had the power to prevent rice from growing. The villagers were reluctant to let the rice leave the territory where the spirits reigned. The villagers believed that they could give away some of the rice, but if they sold it the spirits would be angry and would withhold power from the rice fields.

The economist did not offer a way for the villagers to address the spirits. In his world view, economics was a factual enterprise. In contrast, peace with the spirits was a religious problem. Yet without addressing the relationship between the people and the spirits, the economist was powerless to address what the people perceived as their basic economic problem: the influence of the spirits on the distribution of their rice.

In another village, explains Eric de Rosny in *Healers of the Night*, a merchant opened a business and became somewhat wealthy. He had a simple business strategy: he sold his merchandise at prices below those of the competition. He compensated his lower profits by a higher volume of individual sales. As his business grew, the merchant hired seventy people to work in his shop, and increased his volume of sales and profits accordingly.

The people in the village saw the success of the business as a mystery. How could someone make money by selling merchandise so inexpensively? To people who believe spirituality is the direct cause of everything, a form of sorcery was the only answer. It was not only an economic or physical issue, but a spiritual one.

The victims of this sorcery believe that they live in dimensions of reality that differ from those of the rest of the population. They are poor, while others are rich; they are powerless, while others are powerful; they have a captive existence, while other people are liberated. What is good news to these people?

How does the worldly philosophy address spiritual issues?

In this chapter, we will examine how economic principles affect holistic Christian development. We will see the role of economics in empowering people, and focus on small enterprise development (SED) to illustrate how people can be empowered to raise the quality of their lives by participating in their economies. I believe that economics transcends the spiritual-physical dichotomy because it has an inevitable impact on the realization of *shalom* in a culture. God's concern for justice in *shalom* erases the dichotomy that separates economics from spiritual issues, and makes economics intrinsically spiritual.

Economics is commonly defined as the study of producing, distributing and consuming limited resources. When the early economists first developed the concepts of modern economics, people dubbed them the *worldly philosophers*. People separated economics from spiritual issues as they struggled with the seemingly mundane tasks of understanding how they could produce and equitably distribute resources in a particular society.

The early economists, like contemporary ones, addressed such issues as whether wealth could be created or simply redistributed. They calculated the amount of savings, investments and spending that societies required to prevent recessions and depressions. They also struggled with the morality of compensating for losses on one product by raising prices on other products, a practice that theologians and moral philosophers condemned.

Early economists also struggled to find ways of empowering people to get their just portion of economic resources in a particular economy. Adam Smith and Karl Marx represent the extremes of economic thought. Adam Smith, whose economic principles gave birth to capitalism, said *the invisible hand of capitalism* would distribute resources equitably as individuals pursued their self-interest. Karl Marx saw things differently. He believed capitalism undercut the interests of the poor majority for the benefit of the wealthy few.

Missing in both philosophies was a spiritual principle around which to organize the discipline. Economists would accept the problem of empowering the woman I mentioned earlier who wanted to get a sewing machine. Yet they would not think this problem has a spiritual nature. They would have little to say to the villagers who were afraid to sell their rice, and the victims of sorcery that Eric de Rosny wrote about were beyond their world view.

What philosophy of economics results in *shalom*?

Does the Bible favor one economic system over another? I believe the Bible endorses any economic system that considers *shalom*. What the Bible emphasizes about economic and other similar systems is that they are fallen but they also participate in God's redemptive work through Christ. The central issue, then, is discerning which system most effectively serves its constituents.

Economic statements throughout the Bible do not make physical or spiritual distinctions. Instead, the concern for physical welfare is intensely spiritual. The Old Testament prophets—envisioning a society organized around the cooperative nature of the kingdom of God—summoned people to seek justice, encourage the oppressed, defend the orphan and plead for the widow (Isa. 1:17). People were not to strip the fields of the harvest or pick the vineyards bare (Lev. 19:9-10). They were to leave something for the poor and disenfranchised.

The prophet Ezekiel, in his concern for economic justice, cited the destruction of Sodom as an economic problem. In his view, the collapse of that city was due to the refusal of its inhabitants to care for the poor and needy (Ezek. 16:49). Ezekiel would have been stunned by the modern reader's interpretation of the Genesis account of Sodom's destruction as spiritual, and his account as physical. Such a distinction would not have occurred to Ezekiel because he saw the unjust distribution of resources as an intensely spiritual problem.

In the New Testament, Jesus endorsed the cooperative nature of *shalom* that the prophets proposed concerning the distribution of material resources. He instructed people to live through God's daily provision (Matt. 6:11), he told the rich young ruler to give away all that he had (Mark 10:21), and he said it was easier for a camel to go through the eye of a needle than it was for a rich man to enter the kingdom of God (Mark 10:25). Evidently, the people whom Jesus saw accumulating resources did not express *shalom* in their communities.

What do these teachings tell us about the distribution of resources in our society? Do they show the Bible favoring one economic system over another?

If we do not see economics in a holistic sense—erasing the physical-spiritual dichotomy and recognizing the spirituality of justice—the biblical teaching on the distribution of resources creates a huge dilemma for us. We have to explain why Jesus put so much emphasis on the stewardship of our resources if it is incidental to our well-being.

Christians from modern economies have coped with this dilemma by debating the tensions between capitalism and communism. They discussed whether the Bible endorses the self-interest of capitalism or the social interests of communism. Is the invisible hand of capitalism, as some Christians suggest, really "God's providential structuring of our economic and social life?"[2] Does the sharing of property in Acts suggest that community welfare takes precedence over individual interests (Acts 4:32)?

The first round of the debate is over. Capitalism, whether or not it is the providential hand of God, won; Marxism and socialism lost. We can speculate on whether capitalism, because of its competitive nature, will eventually defeat itself. Yet working toward transforming and modifying the competitive nature of capitalism to reflect the cooperative nature of *shalom* is a more productive task.

Economics as the distribution of power

Defining economics as the production, distribution and consumption of limited resources is acceptable for our purposes, but it has a major flaw. It limits the items of economic concern to those that have measurable values. It correctly recognizes food as an economic resource because we can measure the value of food in any economy. But it does not recognize resources that do not have a measurable value—such as power, in the sense that some people have it and others do not.

This flaw is unfortunate because power is central to economics. In this sense, power is morally neutral, but receives a moral value by how people use it. It can assist or impede the sense of *shalom* in a community. It is the main ingredient that separates the rich from the poor. While people with economic resources get power, the inverse is more often true. People with power in a culture get economic resources. The economic needs of people who are powerless invariably go unmet.

When Christians engage in economic development, they are attempting to empower people. Like the victims of sorcery I mentioned earlier, the situations of the poor render them powerless to use their natural and acquired talents and skills effectively.

This sense of powerlessness is a primary characteristic of poverty. Its effects are crucial to the economic aspects of holistic Christian development, but they are not limited to economics. They pervade the other aspects of our personalities. In the individual, power promotes self-esteem and self-control. It is also "the medium through which we discern our human hunger for the divine dignity that God intended to be our divine birthright as children created in his image."[3]

To paraphrase Joe Remenyi, economic or any other type of development that does not empower people is not development at all. The effective use of power nurtures our self-confidence, and enhances our relationships with others and, ultimately, with God. It cultivates our emotional, intellectual and spiritual growth. Professionally, it "overcomes our feelings of inadequacy by increasing our confidence."[4]

The gap between the rich and the poor is a power gap that creates a dual economy in individual cultures. Dual economies occur when there is no bridge, such as a middle class, connecting the rich and the poor. They create situations where the poor must compete with the rich for essential commodities. This situation creates prices that are extremely expensive for the poor, but somewhat inexpensive for the rich.

Dual economies put an extraordinary portion of total resources in the control of the wealthy. In developing economies, the wealthiest 20 percent of the population controls as much as 60 percent of a nation's income.

In Asia, this means that the wealthiest 20 percent receive almost nine times as much income as the bottom 20 percent. In Africa, the wealthiest 20 percent receive more than 16 times as much as the poorest 20 percent, and in Latin America they receive in excess of 20 times as much.[5] This economic situation is roughly analogous to North Americans who earn $10,000 per year competing for essential commodities with people who earn $200,000 per year.

While these figures show that poverty and wealth are different ends of the same economy, they make the lives of the poor profoundly different from those of the rich. A wealthy few live in palaces surrounded by the shacks of the masses. The destitute dig crumbs from the trash heaps of the wealthy. The poor seek a few buckets of clean water to keep themselves alive while the wealthy use filtered water for their swimming pools and golf courses.

Meeting the just demands of the poor

The economic concerns of holistic Christian development are: 1) What are the just demands[6] of the poor?; and 2) when does meeting the self-interests of wealthy individuals become harmful to the community's welfare?

An ideal answer to these questions might be: "Self interest becomes detrimental to a community when the competitive nature of capitalism becomes more appealing to the people in that community than the cooperative nature of *shalom*, preventing the poor from getting the basic needs of life." But in a more pragmatic world, economics that is concerned with *shalom* seeks to insure that the luxuries and excesses of the rich do not jeopardize the just demands of the poor.

On an international level, economics should wrestle with the justice of transferring resources from poor nations to pay the interest and expenses on debts to rich nations. It should ask if the aid that caused the debts has a beneficial effect on the poor, or if, as a Somali friend told me, "Foreign aid is like giving a naked man a hat."

Economics from a Christian perspective also recognizes the validity of Julius Nyerere's frustration. The former president of Tanzania protested the amount of money foreign debt was draining from his country's economy by asking, "Shall we let our people starve so we can pay our debt to the rich nations of the world?"

An economic philosophy concerned with *shalom* asks why economies cater to the luxuries and excesses of the rich while not satisfying the just demands of the poor for the basic needs of life. In any economy, the luxuries of the rich prevent the poor from getting the necessities of life, because economies do not cater to needs—they cater to demands. All over the world, the rich have the power to demand where societies invest the resources of their economies.

In developed economies, the problem of economics meeting demands instead of needs manifests itself, among other ways, in housing. The market's demands set the housing prices. People on either end of the housing market—those who buy expensive or inexpensive housing—can demand that prices go up or down depending on the availability of housing. The rich can price the poor out of the market; the poor can organize themselves to make low-cost housing economically viable.

In developing economies, the laws of demand affect such necessities as food. An East African proverb says: "The stomach is the most difficult container to fill." A survey completed by my students in East Africa proved the truth of this proverb.

The students compared the prices of food in the markets to the incomes of people on the lower and upper ends of the dual economy. The price of one chicken, approximately $2.00, is equal to 3 percent of a monthly wage on the lower end of the dual economy. The price of a kilogram of beef was equal to 6 percent of a monthly wage of a low income household. If people on the higher end of that country's dual economy had to pay comparable percentages of their income for chicken and beef, a chicken would cost $32.00 and beef would cost $64.00 per kilogram.

Solutions to bridging the gap between the rich and the poor

How does economics bridge the gap between the rich and poor? Economists have proposed several solutions.

One solution is to control the prices of commodities to make them more affordable to the poor. This solution, as shown by the recent collapse of the Soviet economy, invariably fails. People create a black market with inflated prices for the commodities the government exercises price controls over. These commodities, then, become available only to the people who can afford to pay inflated prices.

For example, in one African economy, the government controlled the price of sugar to approximately fifty cents per kilogram. A businessman refused to provide sugar for that low price, and made it available only to people who could pay the black market price of $3.00 per kilogram. This situation made the poor worse off than they were before the government implemented price controls.

A second solution admits that economic benefits disproportionately benefit the rich, but asserts that benefits trickle down from the rich to the poor. Supporters of this solution base it on the fallacy that the poor are empowered to the extent that they participate in the systems that empower the rich. Participating in these systems invariably consists of using the benefits of upgraded airports, new roads, the restructuring of international debt, and improved educational institutions.

This solution seriously fails because of its inability to remove the obstacles that disempower the poor. The hunger, illiteracy and exploitation that the poor experience prevent them from taking advantage of any benefits that might trickle down to them.

A third solution—a variation on the trickle-down theory—is worth mentioning. It states that people should pay higher prices for products that the poor produce.

The production of coffee in Kenya is a good example for illustrating this solution. Coffee growers pay the coffee pickers in Kenya approximately $1.50 per day. The reasoning behind the third solution states that a rise in coffee prices would enable the coffee pickers to earn more income—perhaps $1.75 per day.

The problem with this solution is that the price of coffee does not determine the wages of the coffee pickers. While accumulated expenses set the lowest acceptable prices for any product, there is no direct connection to the prices of goods and the expenses of producing them. Prices are based on what people who purchase particular goods will pay for them.

Therefore, profits do not trickle down to affect wages. Instead, the supply and demand of labor in the Kenyan labor market determines the wages of the coffee pickers. Unfortunately, the abundant supply of labor in Kenya depresses the demand. People who have only their labor to sell in a surplus labor market will work for a meager income simply because they have no power in the economic system.

Small enterprise development contributes to empowerment

Of the several approaches economists use to empower people economically, the remainder of this chapter will focus on involvement in small enterprise development. Small enterprise development (SED) has gained considerable attention in recent years because it effectively empowers the poor to upgrade their living standards. It is one approach that we can incorporate effectively into holistic Christian development.

SED projects support the cooperative principle of holistic Christian development because they generally fit the categories of *good work* defined by E.F. Shumacher. "They give people opportunities to utilize and develop their faculties; they enable people to overcome their inborn self-centeredness by joining with other people in a common task, and they bring forth the goods and services needed by all of us for a decent existence."[7] These qualities assist the realization of both individual and corporate empowerment that *shalom* represents.

The key to successful SED projects lies in identifying services and products that are necessary—but expensive or unavailable—for increasing a community's quality of life. These are usually not the staples of life, but are one or two steps above the staples—such as prepared foods, tailoring services, and crafts.

Someone in a developing culture made peanut butter with a meat grinder after realizing the demand for peanut butter was one step above the demand for peanuts. Other people purchased sewing machines to become tailors after realizing that an increase in the standard of living created a demand for more clothing.

Well-managed SED projects produce impressive success stories. In an African Islamic culture, where economically vulnerable women carry the burden of family support, a group of women developed a cooperative to start a tree nursery. A voluntary organization gave an initial grant to purchase supplies, and the women donated a few hours of their time each week to water, weed and sell the trees. The project provided a good source of cash and a way for the women to become more independent of the social and religious structures that oppressed them. It also provided the community with an essential product.

In *Where Credit Is Due*, Joe Remenyi cites the small enterprise development program of World Vision Sri Lanka as a "spectacular success."[8] The following hallmarks of the program complement the cooperative principles of the kingdom of God that *shalom* symbolizes.

The people based the program on close cooperation with existing social, institutional and cultural structures. It was also village-based, and run entirely by village personnel. And they protected the project from corruption by requiring the villagers to hold regular open meetings to announce successful loan applicants, to record repayments, and to discuss other related issues.

An SED project in a nomadic culture in the Sahel loaned goats, sheep and donkeys to pastoralists after their herds were destroyed. The families who participated in the program had to be poor, of good character, solid members of the community, and willing to participate in other project activities. Each participating family that was loaned livestock agreed to repay these loans within three years with the offspring of the livestock. Eighty percent of the participating families in one location no longer needed assistance after they increased their herds and repaid their loans.

World Vision Colombia invented the word *coopdiaconia* (from the Greek word *diaconia*) to express the principles of its SED program. *Coopdi-*

aconia combines the concepts of community, cooperation, and servant-hood. In an article in *Together*, Augusto Libreros explains that *"coopdiaco-nia's* fundamental reason for being is to give testimony to the Lord Jesus Christ and to his work of love and restoration of the whole person."[9]

A primary principle of *coopdiaconia* is valuing work as liturgy and worship. This perspective adds social and mental blessings to the material benefits of work. It transforms the market economy's competitive nature into one of cooperation and service by confronting the temptation to pursue excessive profits or to turn work into an instrument of oppression.

In an economy where the wealthiest 20 percent control 53 percent of the income and the poorest 20 percent scramble for 4 percent of the income,[10] *coopdiaconia* helps to close the gap of powerlessness that puts the poor and rich in apparently different dimensions of life. *Coopdiaconia,* an expression of "God's plan of grace, love and restoration,"[11] reflects *shalom.* To this extent, holistic Christian development moves economics out of life's physical dimension by acknowledging that the values expressed in the process are valid expressions of God's kingdom on earth.

NOTES

1. *Comparative advantage* is an economics term that states that economies should produce goods that they are most proficient at producing, export the surplus of these goods, and import goods that they are less proficient at producing.

2. John Jefferson Davis, *Your Wealth in God's World: Does the Bible Support the Free Market?* (Phillipsburg: Presbyterian and Reformed Publishing Co., 1984), p. 7.

3. Richard J. Foster, *Money, Sex and Power: The Challenge of the Disciplined Life* (New York: Harper and Row, 1985), p. 208.

4. Ibid., p. 211.

5. Joe Remenyi, *Where Credit Is Due: Income-Generating Programmes for the Poor in Developing Countries* (London: Intermediate Technology Publications, 1991), p. 4.

6. *Demand* is the quantity of a particular commodity that people will buy at a particular price. The term indicates that economies are based on what people demand rather than what they need. Sometimes demands and needs are consistent, though often the demands of the rich prevent the needs of the poor from being met. In such situations, because economies meet demands instead of needs, the needs of the poor go unmet until these needs become demands.

7. E. F. Shumacher, *Good Work* (New York: Harper and Row, 1979), p. 118.

8. Remenyi, p. 82. The World Vision project cited by Dr. Remenyi is actually a credit-based income generation project—a type of small enterprise development project.

9. Augusto Libreros, "Expressing Christian Solidarity," *Together*, Vol. 30 (April-June 1991): 14.

10. World Bank, *World Development Report 1991: The Challenge of Development* (New York: Oxford University Press, 1991), p. 262.

11. Libreros, p. 14.

EIGHT

Healing:
Myth, magic or science?

God did extraordinary miracles through Paul.
Handkerchiefs and aprons
that had touched him were taken to the sick,
and their illnesses were cured and the evil spirits left them.
Acts 19:11-12

. . . Jesus put his fingers into the man's ears.
Then he spit and touched the man's tongue.
He looked up to heaven and with a deep sigh said to him,
"Ephphatha!" (which means, "Be opened!").
At this, the man's ears were opened,
his tongue was loosened and he began to speak plainly.
Mark 7:33-35

"Which is easier:
to say, 'Your sins are forgiven,'
or to say, 'Get up and walk'"?
Luke 5:23

A ROMAN CATHOLIC MISSION has been somewhat successful in planting a church in a folk Islamic community in East Africa. In contrast to other Christian missions that could not build a fellowship beyond a few initial converts in the region, the Catholic mission's fellowship comprises a cross section of the population.

We can credit the Roman Catholic mission's growth to, among other reasons, the similarities between the roles of the priests and the spiritual leaders of the Islamic community regarding healing and health. The medical mission's staff of priests and nuns expressed God's healing power through modern medicine and through prayer, confession, and the redemptive power of the communion elements. Because the people made no distinction between natural and supernatural healing, they did not separate the roles of the priests as spiritual leaders and healers. The priests facilitated God's healing power in specific situations through culturally relevant media. Their healing practices did not create a distinction between physical and spiritual healing.

Instead, the presence of the spiritual leaders—in the absence or presence of medical personnel—affirmed that God was present in the healing process. This holistic approach to medical treatment—integrating the physical and spiritual aspects of healing—enabled converts to Christianity to transform their indigenous models of healing and health to a model that people perceived as Christian.

Healing in these Islamic and Roman Catholic communities was similar to the events recorded in Acts 19:11-12. Through the Eucharist, the priest provided the sufficient sense of harmony between the environment's physical and spiritual elements that the people believed was necessary for healing. The Eucharist was the dynamic equivalent—both culturally and spiritually—of *baraka*, the manifestation of divine power in Islamic cultures. Depending on one's perspective, *baraka*—like the Eucharist—is either myth or magic.

Defining myth, magic and science

In this chapter, we want to examine the nature of healing in terms of myth, magic, and science. We will find that—despite the methods used—healing, to a large extent, is mythological. Because of the mythological nature of healing, the focus of holistic Christian missions is not to dispel the mythology, but to transform it. Holism challenges the idea that healing is either natural or supernatural, an idea that has either never gained credibility or is losing the credibility it once had.

Healing does not fit comfortably in either box of Figure 8.1 on page 127. People who are ill are unwilling to eliminate the possibility that God heals through natural or supernatural means. The problem for medical practice in holistic Christian development is transforming the either-or to both-and. Healing is both natural and supernatural because God is the Creator of the physical media that heal, and he uses healing as part of his redemptive work in creation.

The question healing raises in holistic Christian development is understanding the relationships in the healing process between myth, magic and science. Before addressing these relationships, defining the terms is important. What do myth, magic and science mean?

We can define magic as manipulating powers to realize particular changes. It is not merely slight of hand, but the recognition that some

Figure 8.1   The spiritual-physical dichotomy

Spiritual (supernatural, sacred, values, private)	**Physical** (natural, secular, facts, public)
Theology Religion Ethics Christian Education Healing?	Physical Sciences Social Sciences Economics Education Politics Healing?
(Evangelism)	*(Development)*

people can control non-physical powers to effect change. In magic, people are in control, and their success or failure depends on whether they meet their particular goals. Scripture forbids the use of magic (Ezek. 13:20; Rev. 21:8, 22:15).

Science, on the other hand, is the systematic pursuit of knowledge. Its concern is with observing relationships between varying events, proposing explanations for these relationships, and testing the validity of the explanations by evaluating their ability to predict future events. Reliability is central to science, and it is expressed in terms of the probability that a particular outcome will result from the application of specific methodology.

For lack of a better term, I am using the word myth in contrast to magic. By myth I mean "the nonempirical reality and activity of God in an empirical context."[1] In this sense, myth is a positive term. It communicates the feeling of awe that people experience when they realize the power of God through a given medium. In Christianity, this medium can be a story, parable, proverb, the Eucharist or a healing.

Unfortunately, the word myth has developed negative meanings in modern cultures and languages. The term comes from the Greek word *mythoi*, which simply means "stories." It came to mean "false stories" when early Christians separated what they saw as the true stories of Christianity from the untrue stories of Greek, Roman, and other religions. We continue to use myth to say something is false.

But the true-false dichotomy misses the point of myth. Communicating a mysterious, powerful truth in a particular culture is a better use of the term. Myths are culturally relative. The Greek and Roman stories that the early Christians saw as false—if they were false—undoubtedly had power in their respective cultures. They did not have power for the early Christians, but they had power for the Greeks and Romans.

Actors, athletes and musicians have become the mythological figures of our culture. They have the power to change how people think and behave. After Magic Johnson, an American basketball star, became HIV positive, he committed himself to campaigning for "safe sex." His commitment to this campaign put him on the list of the most admired people in the nation. People everywhere hailed him as one of a few public figures who could influence how others perceived their vulnerability to the AIDS virus.

We often miss the point of myths because we want to turn them into theology, but myths and theology are separate sides of religious expression. If we think of religion as a coin, myth comprises one side and theology comprises the other side. Theology seeks truth with questions; mythology reveals truth through stories, rituals and events. In the words of Joseph Campbell: "Theology gets caught up too often in explaining the meaning of life rather than seeking the experience of being alive."[2]

We are likely to miss the experience of our faith if we do not balance theology and mythology. If we read the New Testament with theological questions and ignore its mythology, we limit our ability to see the power of God revealed in it. The healings of Jesus, for example, were mythological in that they motivated both the people he healed and the observers of his healings to experience the power of God.

Healing continues to serve that purpose. If people in any culture are so inclined, they will see the power of God revealed in healing. After Jesus healed the paralytic (Luke 5:17-26), "Everyone was amazed and gave praise to God (vs. 26)." The Pharisees, though, whose theological assumptions separated them from the culture of the masses, did not see God's power in the healing incident.

Separating myth from magic

Since healing in various cultures apparently takes place through myth and magic, holistic Christian development's task is discerning how Christianity can reveal God's power through healing without communicating a sense of magic.

This task has led modern Christian missions to keep medicine on the natural side of the natural-supernatural dichotomy. It has done so by elevating Western, scientific medicine to a supracultural level, making it the preferred—if not the exclusive—domain of Christian medical missions. From a Western point of view, the marriage of Christianity and

Western medicine protected and prevented Christian missionaries from embracing magic and non-Christian spiritual powers in their medical treatment. But this marriage divorced people with primal world views from their indigenous ideas of healing and health. It drove a wedge into their view of the nature of creation, separating the physical order from its spiritual impetus.

This separation caused several writers to challenge the primacy of Western medicine in Christian missions. These writers are attempting to dispel the belief that medicine based on Western science, in contrast to traditional healing practices, is somehow more acceptable to Christianity's spirituality than traditional methods. They argue that God's redemptive power transcends cultural preferences and is apparent in a variety of healing traditions.

J. A. Stromberg, formerly of the World Health Organization (WHO), supports the use of traditional medicine in Christian missions. He transcends the categories that contrast traditional with Western medicine by defining the former as:

> . . . the sum total of all the knowledge and practices, whether explicable or not, used in diagnosis, prevention and elimination of physical, mental or social imbalance, and relying exclusively on practical experience and observation handed down from generation to generation, verbally and in writing . . . The physical and spiritual aspects of life are stressed, thus giving new dimensions to man and a system of health care by which he maintains his health.[3]

Stromberg maintains that traditional health care treats the entire person, not just the symptoms, and believes it is a resource that should be brought into primary health care. Other writers, realizing that traditional medicine is finding a place in the modern world, commend it for using a holistic approach to health. Traditional health care emphasizes the relationship between the emotional, physical, cultural and spiritual aspects of health.

In *African Culture and the Christian Church*, Aylward Shorter defends the merits of traditional medicine by dispelling the assumptions that traditional healers are witches or "witch doctors." The term "witch doctor" is a misnomer. It suggests "to the uninitiated that the doctor himself is a witch."[4] In many indigenous African languages, the word for the traditional medical practitioner is "reconciler."[5]

Witch doctor is a lamentable term coined by Westerners who could not tell the difference between the people who cause illnesses and those who cure it. Although witches frequently call themselves traditional healers, or doctors, doctors themselves are not witches. They may perform retaliatory rituals, but their primary concern is finding the root cause of illness, and eliminating it.

In the milieu of African cultures, traditional healers try to identify the problems in the network of personal, communal, physical and spiritual relationships that create illness. According to Stromberg, traditional healers catalyze the hope of society. In this regard, their value is preventative, not just curative.

Traditional healers keep people healthy by facilitating "hopes for good health, protection and security from evil forces, prosperity and good fortune, and ritual cleansing when harm or impurities have been contacted."[6] They treat the whole person by reestablishing the sense of personal harmony that is jeopardized when someone experiences illnesses, misfortune and bad luck.

Discerning the legitimacy of traditional healing

Christian medical practitioners can, with some reservations, affirm the legitimacy of traditional practices. The sense of wholeness that accompanies healing in traditional medicine is consistent with the New Testament concept of *soteria*. New Testament authors used the word to describe both salvation and healing. *Soteria* is an aspect of *shalom*. It is "basically and essentially healing, the reestablishment of a whole that was broken, disrupted, disintegrated."[7]

The New Testament would affirm the nature of traditional healing by not making a distinction between physical and spiritual healing. Yet the legitimacy of the healing rests in a world view that dictates how we address the sources of healing. The Western, theistic world view generally discounts indigenous sources of healing. Westerners are reluctant to support healing apart from scientific medicine. They assign healing to the physical side of the physical-spiritual dichotomy, and the intervention of spiritual powers in the physical realm causes apprehension.

In contrast, the primal world view sees the spiritual sources of healing in terms of relationships that involve both the spiritual and physical realms; the two cannot be separated. The concern of traditional healing is with the natures and powers of the spirits. Are the spirits strong or weak, good or bad? Are they spiritually neutral?

The question for Christians is, "Can we transform or integrate a culture's mythology into a holistic world view, one that does not see healing as either scientific or spiritual, but credits all healing to God's redemptive work in creation?"

The need for a holistic world view in medicine became apparent to me during a trip to West Africa. I heard about a black stone that effectively treated snake, scorpion and insect bites. The first person who told me about the stones was an indigenous Christian who condemned the practice. He believed the healing the black stone facilitated relied on indigenous spiritual powers that Christians should not use.

After that conversation, I met some Western Christian missionaries who used the stones because they believed the stones effectively treated bites. "If you put the stones on the bites and bandage the bites," they told me, "the wound will heal. After the wound heals, you can soak the stones in milk and use them again."

The missionaries claimed the stones had no spiritual power. Instead, the stones caused a chemical reaction that aided healing. They recommended that every first aid kit should have one.

Who was right? Was the indigenous Christian leader correct in assuming the treatment from the stones had a spiritual basis? Or were the missionaries correct in assuming the treatment was completely physical?

Within the context of their differing world views, they were both right. The world view of the Western Christian missionaries did not think the chemical reactions caused by the stones had spiritual origins. The healing power of the stones was merely a physical reaction. Their mythology of healing did not enable them to see God tangibly revealing himself in the healing process.

The African Christian leader, on the other hand, could not imagine healing apart from a spiritual basis. He summarily dismissed the methods of traditional healing as part of non-Christian spirituality without giving thought to how Christ's redemptive work could transform these methods.

Holism bridges the gap between these two understandings of healing by determining if the local spirits are responsible or if they are simply getting credit for what God makes possible through his creation. In this situation, the healings the black stones aided seem effective despite spiritual perceptions, making them independent of the local spirits. The stones apparently work despite the spiritual convictions of the users, showing that God the Creator endowed them with some properties that aid healing.

Transforming myths

In many situations, healings are not spiritually neutral. People who facilitate healing through indigenous spirits and religions can no longer effect it if they change their mythology or theology.

For example, some Muslims in the different Islamic Sufi orders are known for rituals that aid healing. I once visited the grave of a famous sheikh, and noticed a key hanging from the tombstone. When I asked why the key was there, my host told me it symbolized the power of the sheikh to unlock the closed womb of sterile women.

My host added that the power of the deceased sheikh works only if a person stays in the village. People who leave the village for the city cannot use the power of the sheikh even if they return to the village. Apparently, the mythology of the people who leave the village changes. Either they no longer have contact with indigenous healing spirits, or they transform their mythology and discontinue belief in the sheikh's power after exposure to urban life. Perhaps they become secularized, modernized or influenced by other religions.

In other situations, the culture's mythology undergoes transformation after religious, cultural or residential changes. In Zaïre, an illness broke out in a community shortly after its people became Christians. The missionaries distributed medicine to the new converts, but ran out of it before the people were cured. The missionaries gathered the people together to pray that God would bridge the gap between the physical and spiritual aspects of creation by providing medicine before the illnesses got worse.

Unlike the missionaries, the Zaïrians did not see a gap between physical and spiritual healing. They affirmed the idea of praying, but thought that praying for God to deliver the medicine was taking a step backward. They believed God could heal them without the medicine. As they prayed for the delivery of the medicine, they also prayed for healing. When the medicine arrived, it was no longer needed—the people were healed.

The Zaïrians converted to Christianity and transformed their mythology in a holistic sense. They always believed in the power of the spirits to heal, and effectively transformed this belief to seeing the power of God in healing. Yet their view of healing changed. They no longer believed that healing was the work of capricious spirits, but now saw it as the evidence of God's grace.

Transforming, redeeming or integrating mythology requires discernment. In discerning the nature of healing, through whatever means, Christians can start by understanding the nature of the healings that Jesus performed. Healing commands significant attention in the Gospels. Contemporary philosophers held a world view that did not believe the body and created matter were worth redeeming or healing. In contrast, Jesus, through healing, affirmed creation's goodness by including all creation in the redemption that the kingdom of God effects.

Why did Jesus heal the sick?

When those of us who are Western Christians look at the teachings of Jesus, we usually miss the point of his healings: we want to understand *how*, not *why*, he performed them. In this manner, we want to transform mythology into science, or magic. It leads us to focus on techniques, asking how we can duplicate them. Do the methods work for us? Are we doing something wrong? Do we have enough faith? Asking if we have enough faith is a short step from asking if God will submit to our will. By doing so, we see God submitting to our faith instead of us submitting to his will.

The more effective approach to transforming mythology is understanding why Jesus healed as he did. The classifications and methods of healing were less relevant to Jesus than his use of healing to proclaim the coming of the kingdom of God. The Gospel of Mark tells of a man who was deaf and mute. Jesus healed this man by putting his fingers in the man's ears and touching the man's tongue with his saliva (Mark 7:33). In another situation, Jesus used mud made from the earth and his saliva to heal a blind man (John 9:6).

Did Jesus need the mud to heal the blind man? From other passages, we find that Jesus healed through the power of his spoken word (Luke 5:23). Jesus probably did not need the mud, but it was important to the man he healed. It fit this man's mythology of healing, affirming a world view that associated healing with the spiritual anointment of some physical element.

Jesus apparently used the mud more for the benefit of the man he healed than for its intrinsic healing power. Jesus could have healed without the mud, as he did in other healing incidents, but he saw no need to challenge the world view of this Israelite.

Yet Western medical practices in primal cultures, for better or for worse, invariably challenge the world views of indigenous people. Christians should interpret medicine within a holistic, Christian world view. This world view does not favor one method of healing over another, but seeks to understand how any method communicates the redemptive power of God.

Spiritual powers and medicine

In Colombia, a boy who worked as a trash picker developed a skin infection. He went to a medical clinic where he received treatment that included a pharmaceutical that looked like salt. The treatment progressed well, then the infection reappeared.

When the medical personnel examined the child to find why the infection reappeared, they learned the boy's mother had stopped giving him the medicine. She was convinced that someone who was performing sorcery on her son was causing the infection.

The medical personnel did not tell the boy's mother how God's power was manifest in the medicine in a way that made sense to her. Therefore, they could not convince her that something other than sorcery was causing her son's illness. She did not make a distinction between physical and spiritual healing, and had no room in her world view for seeing illness and healing apart from spiritual powers.

Complete treatment of the son's illness had to address his mother's world view. Could the medical personnel expand her view of illness and healing to see that they are spiritual, but separate from sorcery? Illness and healing in this sense, as in the problem of understanding electroshock machines in a primal culture, focuses on God's relationship with creation. It does not separate the physical and spiritual aspects of creation. Instead, it sees all illness as a result of the Fall, and healing as God's commitment to regenerating creation.

In another mission, medical personnel distributed medicine for various illnesses to people who also believed that illnesses have spiritual causes. The indigenous people struggled to make a relationship between the nature of the medicine and the nature of the spirits who caused the illness. They initially assumed the medicine caused the spirits to leave the body, but confusion reigned when they learned that different medicines cured different illnesses.

"Why," they wondered, "can't the same medicine cure all diseases?" The answer to this problem became obvious to them. They concluded that different spirits cause different diseases and illnesses. Therefore, certain medicines have power over particular spirits.

In dealing with this problem, the mission took a step backward. They stopped dispensing medicine because it was frustrating the mission's ability to communicate the Good News of Jesus Christ. This decision makes us wonder exactly how the mission understood the Good News. To people who see spirituality in every physical manifestation of life, the decision to stop dispensing medicine was not good news. Instead, this action communicated the existence of an abstract God who cared little about their pain and suffering.

A step forward would have communicated that the two aspects of creation—the physical and the spiritual—participate in the regenerative work of God. Therefore, the medicine is not casting out spirits—God uses different methods to heal. The medicine does not eliminate the possibility that particular spirits cause illnesses and healing; it extends this belief to see the general effects of sin manifest in creation, particularly in the human body.

A holistic approach to medicine

These examples illustrate the need to interpret health within the indigenous world view, and to shift the interpretation to the context of a holistic world view. This shift challenges Christian medical missions to become more holistic, thus addressing the relationship between the power of God and the powers of medicine.

In her article *African Healer vs. Missionary Physician*, Paula M. Warner wrote that Zaïrian patients attributed their wellness more to personal care than to medicine.[8] This information challenged her to make a shift in her treatment. She concluded that probably 90 percent of all hospitalized patients and the general population in Zaïre sought treatment from both Western missionary doctors and traditional healers.

In this sense, healing was culturally relative. A primary reason why people sought this "dual treatment" was because they believed traditional healing was more holistic than the treatment of the mission hospital. Warner writes that in traditional healing, "the healer becomes the vehicle of restoring broken relationships and thus helps reintegrate the patient into his or her clan and the intimate community. To ignore this basic element of reconciliation is to miss totally the importance of traditional therapy."[9]

Modern medical practitioners are also recognizing the importance of spirituality in their work. Dr. Arthur Kornhaber, a psychiatrist at St. Francis Academy in Lake Placid, N.Y., says: "To exclude God from psychiatric consultation is a form of malpractice."[10]

Herbert Benson, a cardiologist from Harvard Medical School, remains convinced of the healing efficacy of *the faith factor*. "Benson claims that the more 'spiritual' people are—that is, the more they are able to get in touch with a presence that is beyond them yet close to them,' the more likely they are to experience a physiological rejuvenation during meditation."[11] He furthers his conviction in the faith factor by claiming "people who are prayed for heal faster than people who aren't prayed for, even though the patients weren't told that prayers were being said for them."[12]

These convictions are consistent with a holistic approach to medicine. Holism recognizes that wellness results in the harmonization of the physical and spiritual forces of a person's environment. It moves healing from the either-or position of the physical-spiritual dichotomy, and sees all healing as evidence of God's commitment to work redemptively in the fallen creation.

Mahatma Gandhi is credited with saying, "Why should I change my religion because a doctor who professes Christianity as his religion has cured me of some disease?"[13] He had no reason to accept the physician's faith unless the physician's treatment revealed the power of God to facilitate *shalom*, the sense of wholeness that Gandhi himself came to symbolize.

<hr>

NOTES

1. Henry F. Lazenby, "The Mythical Use of the Bible by Evangelicals," *Journal of the Evangelical Theological Society* 34:4 (1991): 485.

2. Belden C. Lane, "The Power of Myth: Lessons from Joseph Campbell," *The Christian Century* (July 5-12, 1989): 653.

3. J.A. Stromberg, *The Christian Concept of Healing*, unpublished paper.

4. Aylward Shorter, *African Culture and the Christian Church* (Maryknoll: Orbis Press, 1973), p. 137.

5. Eric Ram of World Vision International, in a personal discussion.

6. Stromberg.

7. Kenneth L. Luscombe, "Discipleship as a Paradigm for Health, Healing and Wholeness," *Health, Healing and Transformation* (Monrovia: MARC/World Vision International, E. Anthony Allen, *et al*, 1991), p. 60.

8. Paula M. Warner, "African Healer vs. Missionary Physician," *Evangelical Missions Quarterly*, Vol. 26:4 (October 1990): 396.

9. Ibid., p. 399.

10. Kenneth L. Woodward, *et al*, "Talking to God," *Newsweek* (January 6, 1992): 40-44.

11. Ibid., p. 44.

12. Ibid., p. 40.

13. John R. W. Stott, *Christian Mission in the Modern World* (Downers Grove: Inter-Varsity Press, 1975), p. 26.

NINE

The powers:
Working toward their redemption

"When you are brought before
synagogues, rulers and authorities . . ."
Luke 12:11

Everyone must submit himself to the governing authorities,
for there is no authority except that which God has established.
The authorities that exist have been established by God. . . .
For he [the ruler] is God's servant to do you good. . . .
Romans 13:1, 4

For our struggle is not against flesh and blood,
but against the rulers,
against the authorities,
against the powers of this dark world and
against the spiritual forces of evil in the heavenly realms.
Ephesians 6:12

IN THE DUMPS of most major cities throughout the world, people subsist by picking through trash for marketable materials such as plastic, glass, and aluminum. The people who work in the dumps usually live in them, and sell the materials they gather to wholesalers. The wholesalers, in turn, sell the materials to recyclers and manufacturers.

Generally, only a few wholesalers are available in any particular dump to buy the materials. So the people who gather the materials do not have the opportunity to seek higher prices from different buyers. This leaves them without any influence over the prices they receive for their products. This relationship between the gatherers and wholesalers renders the gatherers powerless, and makes the wholesalers the lords of the dumps. The wholesalers decide how little they will pay for the material they buy, condemning the people who live in the dumps to an endless cycle of poverty.

Visits to the dumps, particularly for people from affluent cultures, redefine our ideas of human existence. I would like to say they give new meaning to the expressions "down in the dumps," and "one person's trash is another person's treasure." But the experience of seeing hundreds, and perhaps thousands, of people—men, women and children alike—rummaging through mounds of trash changes our view of who we are.

When I visited the dump in Bangkok, I pondered on the differences between the economic structures that the dump dwellers and I participate in. In one sense, these structures are quite different. The economy that I participate in provides benefits that empower me to stay out of dumps. The Thai economy, however, disempowers the dump dwellers by keeping them in the dump.

In another sense, though, the structures are not so different. In fact, the economic structures in Thailand and the United States are only different expressions of the same global economic structure. The economic and political structures the Thais and I participate in are subsets of the global economic structures in which the Thai dump dwellers participate. This relationship makes the dump dwellers and me distant cousins in global and economic structures.

Is confronting the powers part of our ministry?

The issue that confronts us when we consider a response to the dump economy is deciding how much responsibility we have toward our political and economic cousins. Participants in a conference of Christian holistic development practitioners from a variety of organizations visited a large dump in a major Third World city to address this issue. After their visit, the participants gathered to share their thoughts about designing a Christian ministry to a community of people who lived in the dump.

The responses to the visit were fairly predictable. The development practitioners affirmed the work that missions organizations in the area were doing in the dump. Also, the challenge of developing an adequate strategy to communicate the Good News of Jesus Christ to the people who lived in the dump humbled them. The strategies they discussed included the following components: communicating the Good News, improving the quality of life for the dump residents, and empowering the dump residents to have more control over the prices of their materials.

If the development practitioners had not visited the missions, they could have more easily agreed on how much emphasis they should give to each of the components. But one mission that worked in the dump focused the discussion on the controversies of real life. The people who staffed the mission declared that preaching salvation was their only purpose. While they had a small feeding program, they did not see any redemptive value in this activity. Instead, they fed the children in the community to meet the children's "felt needs."

The felt needs of the community could have also included some sense of empowerment in its relationships with the merchants who purchased the salvaged materials. Yet the mission staff was adamant in their refusal to get political. They refused to entertain any thought that the gospel addressed political or economic issues.

Instead, they tenaciously held to the physical-spiritual dichotomy of Western thought. They believed the Good News of Jesus Christ was limited to the spiritual side of the dichotomy. The mission staff particularly saw politics as a worldly pursuit that would only block the gospel message.

Some conference participants believed the mission staff regarded Christianity as a "fairly private affair, a matter of 'spiritual life' only, which leaves uncriticized and unopposed monstrous evils that crush whole nations,"[1] communities and people. If they granted the existence of these "monstrous evils," the mission staff would not see them as the structures of political, economic or social power that oppress the people in the dump. Instead, these conservative Christians would define monstrous evils as nonmaterial, fallen personalities who hover over the earth in search of people they can attach themselves to by either oppression or possession.[2]

For the mission staff, the power structures the wholesalers grafted themselves into were not evil, but evil could possibly affect the wholesalers themselves. In this sense, evil is personalized and not structural. The staff of the mission would interpret Ephesians 6:12 as referring to the conflict between people and demons who want to possess and oppress people.

Yet the inclination of the mission staff was to let this evil go unopposed because their ministry was not to the wholesalers. Their ministry was to the people living in the dump. The staff believed that Christians have no business confronting the powers in the structures that oppressed the ministry's constituents and that kept these constituents in the dump. The mission staff believed the peace that the Good News brings was the inner, personal serenity their constituents professed when prayer or music enabled them to transcend the oppression of the dehumanizing environment in which they lived.

What is the nature of the powers?

The mission's philosophy catalyzed three major positions held by the holistic development practitioners who attended the conference. The majority agreed with the mission staff. They did not believe the power structures in the community were evil. Instead, they granted that evil forces or beings could influence and possess individuals who held positions in the structures.

If the participants in this group wanted to confront the evil nature of the powers, they could do so by some type of binding, exorcism or encounter. Typically, the person confronting the demons would pray for the demons to flee from the people they are victimizing.

A second group of participants supported the idea that people who held positions of power in the structures made deliberate decisions to oppress the powerless dump dwellers. For these development practitioners, nonmaterial beings that influence people did not embody evil, and evil did not play a role in the structures. Instead, they believed the structures were morally neutral. Evil was only a label for human behavior that the development practitioners saw as morally unacceptable, though the merchants believed their behavior had some level of moral acceptability.

The people in this group would understand that the author of Ephesians 6:12 used metaphorical language. They would argue that we do not have to understand the author's language about the struggle of spiritual growth literally. For this group, the powers could not be exorcised, and the structures did not need to be transformed. Rather, the power of the gospel hinged on changing the behavior of the people who perpetuated the oppression and of those who accepted the oppressive conditions.

A third group of conference participants believed that Ephesians 6:12 referred to the structures. They believed the powers and principalities mentioned in Ephesians were similar to the rulers and authorities mentioned in Luke 12:11. In general, these rulers and authorities are the structures of society. In particular, they are the positions in the dump's structures that give power to the people who hold them.

This group believed the structures dictated the decisions the merchants executed. To this group, the structures took on a personality of their own, primarily because the wholesalers were powerless to change them. This group would argue that the merchants could be professing Christians who felt as powerless in the web of the structures as the residents of the dump.

The people who supported this position argued that the wholesalers used the structures as scapegoats for the decisions they executed.

Because the wholesalers did not believe they controlled their decisions, they refused to take personal responsibility for them. This refusal enabled the wholesalers to attribute their decisions to the laws of a nameless, face-less system that governed the extent of viability each person in the sys-tem experienced. They and the residents of the dump were at the mercy of the powers of the system.

The merchants believed that the laws of supply and demand were examples of the powers that governed the system. The merchants would argue, with some validity, that they could only pay as much for a particu-lar quantity of material as the market forces determined. Therefore, they did not see themselves as perpetrators of an economic system that oppressed the dump dwellers. Instead, they saw themselves as victims of the laws that governed the system.

This third group thought the system even dictated the relation-ships between the people who gathered the materials and the merchants. The structures prevented the merchants and the residents of the dump, whether or not they realized it, from developing personal relationships with each other. The structures also caused the residents of the dump and the merchants to depersonalize their relationships by dehumanizing each other.

The people who lived in the dump dehumanized the merchants, and other people in the structures, by referring to them as *they*. They were part of the system, and they made the rules about how the system worked. They could not be confronted or challenged. If things happened, they were doing them. No one ever asked who they were. No one ever identified who they were, but everybody knew them.

They were an unspoken assumption in any conversation about them. If there was a change in the dump, the people who lived in the dump would ask: "I wonder what they are doing?" If the purpose for a change was not immediately apparent, the question would change to: "I wonder why they are doing that?" They were the powers. The powers did not have names, and the thought of developing relationships with them would never cross the minds of the people they oppressed.

They also had to dehumanize the residents of the dump by refer-ring to them as *the dump dwellers, them,* or *those people*. The use of them, those people, or dump dwellers objectified the people who lived in the dump community. This created the perception that somehow the people who lived in the dump were ontologically different from the people who did not live there. The people who did not live in the dump thought the dump dwellers somehow had an existence that was of a different nature, rather than of a different degree.

For the third group of people, ministering to the dump dwellers required a constructive engagement of the powers inherent in the structures. For this group, the powers and principalities mentioned in Ephesians 6:12 were not metaphors for human behavior or limited to nonmaterial, supernatural beings. Instead, the powers characterized the system of relationships that governed life in the dump. Confronting the powers required the residents of the dump and the wholesalers to realize the nature of the system that was dictating their behavior. Unmasking the powers would enable the oppressors and the oppressed to liberate themselves from the powers.

A structural definition of the powers

The thesis of this chapter leans toward affirming the position of the third group—it defines the powers structurally. This definition does not eliminate the possibility that the powers are nonmaterial personalities that hover in the universe.

Also, this definition does not invalidate the metaphorical use of power language. Instead, it is open to the possibility that the powers, in different situations, are both nonmaterial entities or structures. The value in this interpretation is its recognition that the powers are structures that have an important role in facilitating *shalom* in a community.

Defining powers structurally is important for holistic development because structures account for much of the underdevelopment and oppression that people experience. A structural definition of power recognizes that it is a resource God gives to people, enabling them to fill their positions of authority effectively. In this sense, power is a resource that people who God gave it to have stewardship over. These people are accountable to God, the Creator of the structures, for how they use this resource.

Structural definitions of power recognize that people who have stewardship over power also have fallen natures. Therefore, the power people hold takes on a life of its own. The people who hold power no longer control it; instead, it controls them. Its control causes some people to become oppressors and other people to become oppressed.

Both positions—the oppressors and the oppressed—frustrate the sense of *shalom* that characterizes the kingdom of God. The realization of *shalom* requires their liberation from these positions. As Walter Wink wrote: "If the advanced must die to their positions of egocentricity, the underprivileged must die to their hopelessness, fatalism and acquiescence in their own despoiling."[3]

A structural definition of the powers recognizes that they are "both visible and invisible, earthly and heavenly, spiritual and institutional."[4] They "are 'more,'"[5] they "are not and never have been a mere sum total of the individuals composing them. The whole is more than the sum of its parts. And this 'more' is an invisible Power."[6] The "more" accounts for the fact that although "the powers are established, staffed, and perpetuated by people, they are beyond human control."[7] People get grafted into the powers, and often become what they do not want to be. They lose part of their humanity to become what the powers dictate.

People who are fully possessed by the powers can lose their humanity to the point where they can no longer make morally responsible decisions. Fallen powers dictate the decisions these people make. The people whose decisions are dictated by the powers do not see that the powers exist for the sake of serving people. Instead, they believe what is good for the powers is good for humanity.

Jesus addressed an example of this situation when he reminded the Pharisees that the law—an expression of the powers that governed the people—did not exist for its own sake. The law existed to serve the people: "For the Son of Man is Lord of the Sabbath" (Matt. 12:8).

To an adequate extent, structural definitions of the powers solve the problem of whether redemption also extends to them. Unlike metaphorical or traditional definitions, structural definitions recognize that the powers exist as integral parts of creation, and they participate in Christ's redemptive work. They are among the "thrones or powers or rulers or authorities" (Col. 1:16) that Christ's work reconciles to God.

Addressing the powers

Any strategy to address the powers, principalities, and rulers must begin with the premise that God established and endowed these entities with the authority to maintain order in society. They are God's servants to do good, and Christians must submit to them out of conscientious support for the good they do (Rom. 13:4-5).

Yet the powers, while good, are also fallen. They seek to separate us from the love of God (Rom. 8:38). We find them ruling over the lives of those who live far from the love of God (Eph. 2:2). We find them holding people in servitude to their rules (Col. 2:20), and we find them holding men subject under their tutelage (Gal. 4:3). "The structures which were supposed to be our servants have become our masters and our guardians."[8]

The powers rebelled from their created purpose of enabling people to live genuinely free, human, loving lives by declaring their sovereignty and independence from their Creator. They have "absolutized themselves and they demand from the individual and society an unconditional loyalty."[9] In doing so, "they harm and enslave people,"[10] defeating the very purposes for which God created them.

God is also redeeming the powers. As mentioned earlier, the powers participate in the reconciliation of all things to God through Christ (Col. 1:20). For the Christian community, the issue is how God redeems them. Conservatives tend to believe that God redeems the powers through our support—what we have now is better than what change might bring. Radicals condemn the powers, believing they are destructive. Redemption, for radicals, comes with change. Reformers, in contrast to conservatives and radicals, hope to transform the powers. They see redemption in the hope of restoring the powers to fulfill the purpose for which God created them.

Through submission, God expects Christians to hold these three alternatives together. We submit to the powers simultaneously to condemn, transform and restore them. Initially, this statement sounds contradictory; historically, submitting to the powers has been interpreted as supporting them as they are.

This interpretation is unfortunate because it enhances the conceit of the powers, conferring upon them support that is nearly unconditional for behavior that is often reprehensible. This conservative interpretation of submitting to the powers leaves the Christian community with little ground between supporting and ignoring the powers. It does not give Christians the opportunity to transform or condemn the powers.

Simultaneously condemning, transforming and restoring the powers calls us to distinguish submission from obedience. Scholars usually understand that Scripture passages on submission teach us about obedience. Obedience is defined as unconditionally conforming to the directives of the powers.

Submission, in contrast to obedience, is responding to the powers according to the purposes for which God created them. Submission recognizes that the legitimacy of the powers rests not in what they do, but in their fulfilling the purposes for which God created them. They are to liberate—not oppress—humankind, enabling humanity to lives that are authentically human.

When people submit to the powers, they are either supporting the legitimate authority of the powers or they are accepting the consequences of not supporting the powers. In both situations, Christians are submitting to the powers, but they are not necessarily obeying them.

In many situations, submitting to the consequences of the powers is as legitimate as submitting to the directives of the powers. For example, the crucifixion was the consequence Jesus suffered for submitting to, but not obeying, the powers. The cross was "the political, legally to be expected result of a moral clash with the powers ruling his society."[11] Like all people, Jesus was subject to the powers. "He accepted his own status of submission. But morally he broke their rules by refusing to support them in their self-glorification; and this is why they killed him."[12] In the cross, Christ "disarmed the powers and authorities, he made a public spectacle of them, triumphing over them" (Col 2:15). He exposed "the systems and the principalities for what they actually are—the means to control humans and drag them down to hell."[13]

Toward redeeming the powers

By understanding that the powers exist for humanity instead of humanity existing for the powers, Jesus could live a free and authentic life. He often challenged the powers through such acts as healing people on the Sabbath, primarily because he knew the purpose of the powers was to serve and empower people.

When Jesus healed on the Sabbath—an event people understood as forbidden by the law—he showed that people are responsible for having the law empower, not tyrannize, them. People were to take responsibility for understanding and interpreting the purpose of the law to decide the acceptability of particular behavior. They were not to render the law void, but they were to understand its legitimacy and its ability to empower them.

In most of the world's societies, the powers deny people the basic rights that God had established the powers to provide. The powers exploit laborers, they take advantage of the poor and downtrodden, and they do not defend the widows or orphans. They tend to make powerful people more powerful and the powerless more impotent; the rich become richer and the poor become poorer; the well-fed get fatter and the hungry get hungrier. The powers do exactly the opposite of what God created them to do.

For Christian development work to be holistic, we must work to redeem the powers to the point where they can fulfill their ordained purpose more effectively. We must challenge our tendency to ignore the powers. While we may believe the powers do not affect our work, the people we are attempting to empower cannot live without them.

I have seen development people with marvelous ideas make plans that will prove ineffective because the powers of the community will not support them. The project's constituents will verbally affirm the ideas, but they will not express their tension over what people can plan and what the powers will allow. Their tension is not with agricultural or medical innovations: it is with the powers and principalities that want some personal benefit from the projects.

For example, a medical development project could not get authorization to set up a hospital unless the development agency provided a

Mercedes Benz for the governor of the region. In other situations, development projects could not import supplies unless the people gave a certain percentage of the supplies to the customs officials for their private use.

How is God going to redeem the powers? First, it is important to believe that the powers are not beyond God's redemptive power. "The good news is that God not only liberates us from the powers, but liberates the powers as well."[14] This conviction frees us from having a paranoid view of reality in which we become victims. It will empower us by enabling us to see that the powers are not absolutely evil, but they depend on our prayers for their redemption.

The second step toward redeeming the powers is praying for them. Perhaps they are the enemies Jesus instructed us to love and pray for; possibly they are the persecutors we should bless. In praying for our enemies, we have the opportunity to purify our motives to be more effective in the work we are doing. Through prayer, we also have the opportunity to examine and resist our own temptations for power, and our possible need to identify or to comply with the powers. Through prayer, we liberate ourselves to more fully participate in the redemptive work of God.

Prayer enables us to see God working in us and, through this realization, we can see God working through our enemies. It breaks any power our enemies have over us that prevents us from praying for them and praying for ourselves. Prayer gives us the freedom to experience who we are, and the power to see who our enemies are. Prayer reminds us that Jesus, through the cross, made a spectacle of the powers. Yet he did not alienate them; the powers continue to participate in God's redemptive work through Christ.

The third step in redeeming the powers is meeting them. In seeing the powers face to face, we are likely to unmask them, and find ourselves more empowered to negotiate than we might expect. We can break the idea that the powers are sovereign.

Meeting and unmasking the powers

Once someone brought me to court for a fabricated violation. This court was not part of a judicial system that presumes a person is innocent until proven guilty. Instead, the court assumed guilt to anyone who was charged with a crime or violation. The burden of proof was not on the court, but on the defendant.

When I refused to acknowledge the legitimacy of the charges, the judge asked me what my religion says about responding to people who make false charges against me. I replied that Jesus taught us to love those who persecute us. I affirmed that I believed my accuser was created in God's image, and that he was worthy of the love Jesus taught us to have for our persecutors. Still, I repeated my refusal to acknowledge the validity of the charges that this person brought against me.

After a few more minutes of conversation, the judge's ambivalence toward prosecuting me was apparent. I strongly suspected that he had accepted a bribe from my accuser, and found himself in the predicament of having agreed to a prosecution he could not make. Realizing that he could not close the case, I took the initiative to ease his predicament by walking out of the court.

While driving to the village the next day, I saw my accuser out walking. I stopped, invited him to ride with me, and we chatted about the health and welfare of our families. After a while, he asked if we could meet to talk about the event of the preceding day. We agreed to meet that afternoon. That meeting convinced me that the powers in the village were closer to redemption than they had previously been.

In *Empowering the Poor*, Bob Linthicum wrote of an experience in which the powers were not distributing milk to the children of a Brazilian community. The community understood the problem as a struggle between the powers. This is not an uncommon problem; an African proverb illustrates it well: "When elephants fight, mice are trampled."

Linthicum focused the ensuing discussion on the root of the problem. The powers did not exist for their own benefit, but for the benefit of the people they were serving. He affirmed that the milk did not belong to the powers to do as they pleased. "It's our milk—given to us by the government," Linthicum told the members of the community. "Why should we let them decide how to distribute our milk?"[15]

After realizing the nature of the problem, the community selected representatives to speak to the people in power about the unjust distribution of the milk. In typical fashion, the people in power separated themselves from the powers by blaming the problem on someone else. (This blame perpetuates the idea that the powers exist apart from the people in power because no one in power takes responsibility for the behavior of the powers. This reasoning gives the powers an autonomous existence.)

> Eventually, a public official was influenced to attend a meeting. The public meeting began, and the people quickly began expressing their frustrations. And the health secretary invited all the leaders of the mothers' clubs and the residents' association to speak their mind. And after they were done, he said "Beginning next week, we will begin distributing the milk tickets. I will keep checking with you to be sure the milk is reaching the people."[16]

The people, by meeting the powers, redeemed them. They submitted to the purposes for which God created the powers, condemned the abuse of the powers, and reformed the powers to fulfill their role in the community.

Transforming the powers

This demonstration bore witness to Christ's power to transform the powers in the most profound way. In most cultures the oppressed want to overcome their oppression by being grafted into the structures. They attempt to overcome their oppression by becoming what they hate. In doing so, they lose a part of their humanity; the structures define who they are and the decisions they make.

Christ's power enables people to overcome oppression by addressing the powers without becoming like the powers. The power of Christ liberates people from the temptation of joining the powers that oppress them.

In the crucifixion, Christ made a spectacle of the powers, not by being grafted into them, but by expressing his power in an ontologically different manner from the power of the powers. He submitted to the demands of the powers to the point where they, in attempting to destroy him, lost power over him.

The greatest Christian witness is not in joining the powers; joining them results in people addressing evil by becoming what they hate. It will cause us to interpret the nonviolent teachings of Jesus violently. Instead, the Christian witness to the powers is to transform them by submitting to their ordained purposes, to the point where our submission destroys the corruption of those purposes. This liberates the powers from their corruption and empowers them to fulfill the purposes for which God created them.

The powers mentioned throughout this chapter—those in the dump, the court and the government—are closer to redemption because Christians are willing to work toward redeeming them by submitting to their ordained purposes. God established the powers in the dump to empower the people there to live a more human existence. God established the court to render justice, and the government to distribute community resources more equitably. If Christians do not submit to these purposes, the communities that God established the powers to serve are farther from experiencing the sense of *shalom* that characterizes God's covenant with creation.

NOTES

1. Walter Wink, "Living the Word," *Sojourners* (May 24, 1992): 30.

2. A third alternative is "demonized." It is commonly used to communicate the middle ground between possessed and oppressed.

3. Wink, p. 158.

4. Walter Wink, "All Will Be Redeemed," *The Other Side*, Vol. 28:6 (November-December 1992): 17.

5. Ibid.

6. John Howard Yoder, *The Politics of Jesus* (Grand Rapids: Eerdmans Publishing Company, 1972), p. 146.

7. Walter Wink, *Engaging the Powers* (Minneapolis: Augsburg Fortress Press, 1992), p. 41.

8. Yoder, p. 143.

9. Ibid, p. 146.

10. Ibid.

11. Ibid., p. 132.

12. Ibid., p. 148.

13. Robert C. Linthicum, *City of God, City of Satan* (Grand Rapids: Zondervan, 1991), p. 133.

14. Wink, *Engaging the Powers*, p. 65.

15. Robert C. Linthicum, *Empowering the Poor* (Monrovia: MARC, 1991), p. 27.

16. Ibid., p. 28.

TEN

Holism:
Is it centered, bounded or fuzzy?

[Jesus] told them another parable:
"The kingdom of heaven is like a mustard seed,
which a man took and planted in his field. . . .
yet when it grows,
it is the largest of garden plants and becomes a tree,
so that the birds of the air come and perch in its branches."
Matthew 13:31-32

. . . "I tell you the truth,
whatever you did for one of the least of these
brothers of mine, you did for me."
Matthew 25:40

For the kingdom of God is not a matter of eating and drinking,
but of righteousness, peace and joy in the Holy Spirit.
Romans 14:17

EVALUATING THE HOLISTIC NATURE of Christian development is analogous to evaluating the presence of the kingdom of God. We achieve both through processes instead of acts.

When the disciples asked Jesus about the coming of the kingdom, he answered by comparing it to the process of planting a tree from a seed. At some point in the process the seed grows to become a tree. Before the tree reaches maturity, it is a seedling and a sapling. In each of these immature stages, though, it is still a tree. Likewise, Christian development is holistic and continues to grow toward the fullness of holism, making this movement toward holism a process rather than an act.

The problem Christian development practitioners experience, more often than not, is seeing development as an act, not a process. While the word *development* implies a process, we tend to see it as an act. We usually focus on results—either something happened or it did not happen. We tend to measure things in terms of success and failure. Knowing that we achieved something is more important to us than knowing it is in process. Process communicates a sense of ambiguity that we need to clear up.

Christians thrive on acts, particularly those of us who are influenced by the dichotomies and neat classifications of physical and spiritual, sacred and secular. Figure 9.1 below illustrates these classifications.

But God seems to work in *processes*. For example, sanctification—the first and final purpose of our faith—is a process. Sanctification started with the act of God in the crucifixion, but God continues to work it out during our pilgrimage of faith throughout our entire lives. Like other areas of Christian ministry, we cannot confine sanctification to the upper or lower box of the physical-spiritual dichotomy. It is a holistic concept that transcends our entire being.

People from non-Western cultures also are more likely to think in terms of processes, not acts. The either-or categories that are central to Western thought are less meaningful in other cultures.

Non-Western cultures may have a higher tolerance for ambiguity or have different sets of categories. What we see as either-or in our culture could be both-and in another culture. Other cultures may have less trouble in seeing how *shalom*—because it is both physical and spiritual—makes the boundaries between the two categories meaningless. *Shalom* symbolizes a unified world, not a two-tiered one.

Figure 9.1   The spiritual-physical dichotomy

Spiritual (supernatural, sacred, values, private)	**Physical** (natural, secular, facts, public)
Theology Religion Ethics Christian Education	Physical Sciences Social Sciences Economics Management Secular Education
(Evangelism)	*(Development)*

Evaluating holism in Christian development

Evaluating holism in Christian development, then, is shifting our thinking to see development as a process toward holism that culminates in the realization of *shalom*. In proposing this, I want to focus on evaluating holism in terms of centered sets, bounded sets and fuzzy sets. The conclusion I want to work toward is that we can best evaluate holism through the model of centered sets.

The first assumption in this conclusion is that God's covenant to his people is one of *shalom* that brings harmony to all creation. Effecting *shalom* is not an either-or act. Further, we cannot limit it to salvation in the sense that we separate spirituality from the physical welfare of a person or community. As mentioned in chapter one, *shalom* is not only concerned with people having peace with God—it is shockingly materialistic in its concern for food, clothing and shelter. It symbolizes God's care and concern for the welfare of the entire creation.

The second assumption in evaluating holism is that God's covenant is with communities, not with individuals. The Bible repeatedly addresses spirituality in the context of community. The Lord's Prayer, for example, uses the plural pronouns *our* and *we*. New Testament writers always used the term *saint* in its plural form.

Therefore, holistic Christian development must focus on communities instead of individuals. If a project benefits individuals at the expense of the community's welfare, it is not holistic. One person cannot experience *shalom* in spite of, or at the expense of, the community.

Defining centered, bounded and fuzzy sets

Figure 9.2 on page 154 helps us see the differences between centered, bounded and fuzzy sets.[1] If we ask which of the two figures is closer to God's kingdom, the answer depends on: 1) the set we are using to make the decision, and 2) whether the figures are stationary or moving.

If we look at the diagram from the perspective of a bounded set, Figure B is closer to the kingdom of God than Figure A. If we look at the diagram from the perspective of a centered set, Figure A could be closer, depending on whether it is stationary or moving in a particular direction.

Bounded Sets

Bounded sets define items in terms of acts, positions or categories. They make either-or statements: either something happened or it did not happen. Something or someone is either in or out, left or right, north or south. A long fruit with yellow skin and white pulp fits the criteria for the bounded set of fruit called bananas. Fruit of this description does not fit the criteria included in sets for oranges or any other species of fruit.

Figure 9.2   Who is closer to the kingdom of God?

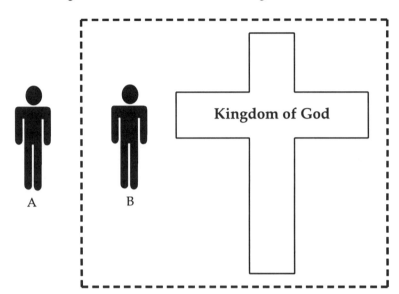

While bounded sets seem distinct, they are culturally relative. I once had a discussion with an African friend about a picture of a camel engraved on a leather bag. When I told him there was a bag with a camel on it on my desk, he was confused. When he found the bag, he corrected my statement, telling me an engraving of a camel was on the bag. The engraving was not a camel. To him, the engraving did not fit in the bounded set of camels—it was part of another bounded set called pictures of camels. In his world view, we could not discuss camels and pictures of camels without making explicit the assumed differences between pictures and the actual animals.

My friend's emphasis on placing the picture of the camel and the actual animal in different sets is analogous to Christians putting the person of Christ and statues of Christ in different sets. People from some Christian traditions are offended at calling an icon Christ. In other Christian traditions, the distinction is less important.

If we look at Christians in terms of bounded sets, they are either in the kingdom or out of the kingdom, saved or unsaved. They may have answered an altar call; they could have been baptized or confirmed, or they might have said the "sinner's prayer." Regardless of how we define the boundary of salvation, they passed over it.

Because bounded sets are static, change and growth are incidental to them. If an object fits into a particular boundary, change within the boundary does not change the identity of the object. A tomato, for example, always fits the criteria of a tomato whether it is growing on a vine or sliced in a salad. Similarly, Christians are Christians as long as they are within the boundaries of salvation. Growth and change do not affect the Christian's identity within the bounded set.

The physical-spiritual dichotomy is the result of bounded sets. If we classified the disciplines that we incorporate into Christian development, they would fit into the bounded sets of physical or spiritual, depending on the issues they address. The disciplines that deal with theology, religion, ethics, values and evangelism fit into the spiritual set. The disciplines that address facts, sciences, or human welfare fit into the physical set.

But the bounded set model clearly breaks down when we see the use of a variety of disciplines in God's redemptive work in creation. This creates the problem of classifying spiritual intervention in the physical set.

Centered Sets

From the perspective of a centered set, Person A in Figure 9.2 may be closer to the kingdom of God than Person B. The deciding factor is the direction in which the persons are facing or moving. If Person A is facing toward the kingdom of God and Person B is facing away from it, Person A is closer to the kingdom, regardless of geographical proximity.

Centered sets, in contrast to bounded sets, are dynamic. Their concern is with processes, instead of acts, criteria or positions. Boundaries are incidental to centered sets; *movement* is the primary concern. In bounded sets, if people are moving toward or away from the kingdom of God, their position at any point in the process loses its meaning. Their location at any given time is less important than the direction in which they are moving. Regardless of its proximity to the kingdom of God, the community moving toward God's kingdom is always closer to it than the community that is moving away from it.

In holistic Christian development, the center of the centered set is the kingdom of God; development participants are the subjects of the set. The evaluation questions ask: Where are the participants of the development in relation to the kingdom of God? Are they moving toward or away from the kingdom? A move toward the kingdom, despite its pace, is a result of experiencing God's redemptive work in creation.

Fuzzy Sets

Fuzzy sets, depicted by the border in Figure 9.2, represent a middle ground between centered and bounded sets. They may help make the transition between conversion as seen in terms of either centers or boundaries. If people who favor centered sets feel comfortable with some type of boundary, a fuzzy set provides a loose boundary.

For people who favor bounded sets, fuzzy sets recognize that some aspects of life, like religious conversion and convictions, are not always expressed in either-or terms. In liturgical Christian traditions, icons fit into fuzzy sets. They are symbols that go beyond representing the saints or Christ, but they are not really saints or the person of Christ. The distinction between these two choices is not always clear. Conversion to Christianity in non-Western cultures also can fit in fuzzy sets.

We could categorize God's intervention in nature as a fuzzy set that exists between the bounded sets of the physical-spiritual dichotomy. The problem we have with this classification is that we seldom find truth in synthesis. A fuzzy set, like a bounded set, divides the physical and spiritual aspects of creation. Holism, however, does not divide the unseen from the seen dimensions of creation. Instead, it separates the nature of the Creator from the nature of creation, causing the fuzzy set to be less than holistic.

Using a bounded set in the task of defining indicators to evaluate holistic Christian development is somewhat simple. We can determine the success of a project by using particular criteria, such as counting converts. We can identify the obstacles to a project's success by defining the reasons why people are not becoming converts. After we identify the reasons for the lack of conversions, we can determine if we can overcome the obstacles.

Evaluating projects according to centered sets determines whether the participants are moving closer to, or further from, the kingdom of God. Centered sets recognize that projects have interdependent temporal and eternal dimensions.

Indicators, therefore, seek to define if the project participants have more peace with the physical and the spiritual realms of creation. Did the project transform the people's fear of the spiritual realm into faith? Did the project empower its participants to take more control over their environments? Is there more economic, social and political justice in the community because of the project? Do they have a higher view of Christianity? Do the people see God's concern for every aspect of their lives? Positive answers to these questions show movement toward the center.

Steps toward the center

The following steps in evaluating the movement of a community toward the kingdom of God are based on the concept of "starting point plus process."[2] This concept complements centered sets because it focuses on a culture's present position in relation to where they came from, and where they are going. It recognizes that holistic Christian development is a process of transformation, and provides markers for mapping that process.

1. Evaluating the attitudes of the community toward the gospel.

Figure 9.3 below shows a community's attitudes toward the gospel in terms of progression. Fundamentalist communities of major religions are perhaps the most antagonistic toward the gospel. African traditional cultures are more neutral, and Latin American cultures have embraced the gospel or are receptive to it.

2. People have a positive attitude toward the gospel

After identifying the community's attitude toward the gospel, the next step is easing a move toward the right end of the scale. We initially do this when the community and the mission come to know each other. The common question asked of missionaries is: "Why are you here?" The answer to that question moves a community toward the positive or negative side of the scale.

When I taught commercial studies in an Islamic culture, I gave considerable thought to why I was there. What impact did my work have on moving the students, and their community, toward the kingdom of God? What did my presence in the culture, the relationships I formed with the students, and the content of my courses say about the kingdom of God? Did questions come up in my classes that I could use to point to the gospel as the answer?

I usually told my students that God had called me to that culture. This statement affirmed their belief that people do things in submission to God. It also raised several questions that challenged the Islamic view of Christianity. The students were devout Muslims who had little regard for Christians. For generations, parents told their children that Christians were infidels who ate pork, drank wine and worshiped three gods. All this led the students to believe that Christians lacked spiritual integrity.

Figure 9.3   A community's progression in its attitude toward the gospel

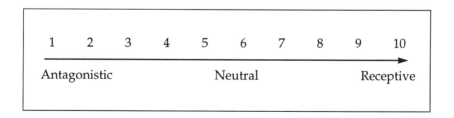

In fact, Muslims believe Christians are apostates of Islam. When Muslims fall from Islam by not practicing the five pillars of the faith, people believe they are becoming Christians. A popular curse in the culture is: "May you die when you are a Christian," wishing people will die in a state of apostasy.

The hostility that my Muslim students held toward Christians had developed over generations. It was not going to disappear within the relatively short time of any missionary presence. Yet as Christians expressed the peace of Christ as they lived among the Muslims, this hostility eased. When I asked a Muslim friend what he would teach his children about Christians, he said he would tell them we are honorary Muslims. This response showed that he was moving closer to the kingdom of God by recognizing the integrity of Christians, if not Christianity.

3. People have a positive attitude toward those who convert to Christianity

One of the greatest obstacles to holding a Western, individual view of conversion to Christianity is a community's attitude toward people who accept another religion. In Western cultures, the physical-spiritual dichotomy relegates religion to the private sphere (Figure 9.1). In this scheme, religious conversion is a personal and private decision that a person makes individually. The family, or another group that a person identifies with, does not have the privilege of interfering with personal decisions.

In cultures where the personal-public dichotomy is not so prevalent, personal decisions, such as religion, are not private or individual. They are public and communal. The community believes that its welfare depends on the welfare of individuals, making personal decisions more communal. In religious matters, individuals do not have the right or privilege to act apart from the community. Those who act apart from the community are subject to social isolation, punishment, and possibly death.

This tension between personal and community decisions poses a severe problem for missionaries. It leads some missionaries to encourage converts to be *secret believers*. Other missionaries encourage converts to leave the community, and a third option focuses on the community's attitudes instead of seeking individual converts. This option trades short-term results for long-term benefits. The decision for either option generally lies in the conviction of individual converts and communities.

4. Making the decision to become a Christian

The presence of Christians in any community usually leads to conversions. The issue that missionaries and converts face is the model of conversion that they and their communities see as legitimate. A Western model emphasizes decisions for individuals to move across the boundaries of salvation. In other cultures, people may prefer conversion and baptism as a community, or not make such either-or decisions. They are prone to avoiding either-or situations, preferring to live with ambiguities.

Recently, mission agencies have paid closer attention to *dynamic equivalent believers*. This model of "conversion" is a point in a transition from a centered to a fuzzy set. It recognizes that in many cultures, conversion does not lend itself to either-or conditions. Instead, it is a progression of movement toward the center, or a step into a fuzzy set. Conversion is not necessarily decisive, but it can be an open-ended process involving tentative decisions to move toward the kingdom of God. The basis for the legitimacy of this model is the idea that the transformation of people and their cultures is a process, not an act.

5. Taking steps toward contextualizing Christianity in a culture

Worship, perhaps more than conversion, is culturally relative. We create environments that are conducive to worship according to the conditions of our culture. In Western cultures, places of worship generally contain such things as pews, music and musical instruments. We wear shoes in the church building and sit on comfortable pews; sometimes we sit next to people of the opposite gender, and we sing. In Islamic cultures, people kneel on carpets; they do not sing; men and women worship in separate sections of the building, and Muslims would never wear shoes when praying.

When we look at cultural worship practices, we frequently ask if they are necessary, and we are prone to discount them if we think they are unnecessary. Instead of discounting these practices, the four steps of critical contextualization that I analyzed in chapter three are useful in evaluating them.

The need for any cultural worship practice depends on where the community is in the process of transformation during their spiritual pilgrimage. For example, when Paul and his associates arrived in Jerusalem, Paul went to the temple to purify himself, and gave a date for when an offering would be made for each of them (Acts 21:26). If we understand Paul's theology correctly, the offering was unnecessary, but apparently it was an important part of Paul's spirituality at that point in his pilgrimage. He was transforming his spirituality from where he was to where God wanted him to be.

6. The community experiences shalom

If holistic Christian development is effective, it will result in an increase in the quality of life for individuals and for the community. This quality of life is achieved in three complementary parts.

a.The middle is redeemed, and people have peace with the spiritual realm

If we contextualize development effectively in primal and modern theistic cultures, the middle will be redeemed. We will not exclude or ignore the personal and impersonal powers between heaven and earth that people believe influence their lives.

Instead, the middle will reflect a view of the spiritual realm that is characterized by *shalom*. As Paul continued the purification rituals at the temple, people with primal world views will undergo a transition enabling them to see the middle as a part of creation participating in the Savior's redemptive work. But gaining this perspective is a process. Fear of the spirits will fade as people from primal cultures experience the peace of Christ, but it will not be extinguished immediately.

We can think of the rites, ceremonies and rituals that appease the middle in terms of their ability to transform worship to the living Savior. In Western cultures, our celebration of Christmas on December 25 and Easter on the Sunday following the first full moon after March 21 reflects the transformation of non-Christian holidays. These holidays were originally Roman holidays that the church integrated into the Christian calendar. Other cultures have harvest rituals, birth celebrations and death rites that Christians can transform into ceremonies that acknowledge God's sovereignty over the lives of people in the culture.

b. Seeing God as the source of innovations and benefits

One of the greatest frustrations of making development holistic is our tendency to see our work as modernizing or Westernizing a culture. If our work does either, it fails. The basis of modernization and Westernization is a secularized idea of unlimited growth. A secular approach to development does not see growth as a means to an end, but as an end itself.

Holistic Christian development's purpose is to implement development by using technology as a tool that aids a culture's ability to experience the progressive revelation of God's kingdom. The issue is not whether people in a culture are growing. The issue is: Are people transforming their culture so they can experience the various dimensions of *shalom*? Are the people experiencing peace with the environment, the community, or the economic life of the community? Are they empowered to have their just demands met? Is there justice in the distribution of resources? Are people's basic needs met, regardless of gender, age and social status?

c. Seeing God as the source of justice

If Christian development is holistic, the community will achieve a sense of justice. Too often, development caters to those who are least in need of justice, bringing more power to those who are already powerful, and enabling the rich to get richer.

The goal of holistic Christian development is to empower the powerless, enabling them to receive a just portion of the benefits of development. Increases in health, education and the quality of life, and decreases in human suffering and in infant and child mortality rates achieve this just portion.

A tale of two missions

Mission agencies A and B operated separate schools in an African Islamic culture. They did not work together, but they had a cordial relationship. One day an official from the Ministry of Education decreed that each mission would have to permit Islamic teachers to teach the Qur'an in the mission schools.

The decree was a setback for both missions, and each responded to it differently. Missionaries from agency A evaluated the effectiveness of their work according to the criteria of a bounded set. They decided the Qur'anic teachers would defeat the purpose for the mission's existence. So they left the country.

Missionaries from agency B decided that leaving the country was a greater threat to their mission than the presence of the Qur'anic teachers in the schools. They were working with spiritually disadvantaged, economically poor and politically powerless people. If the mission left, the people in the community would not experience God's redemptive work in a difficult environment.

Mission B perceived the effectiveness of their mission according to a centered set. They believed their work was to bring *shalom* to the community. They also believed that, despite the obstacles they faced, this work would bear witness to Christ and influence change in the community. Further, their work and presence in the community could move people closer to the kingdom of God, whether or not the community made any steps across arbitrary boundaries.

As the decades passed, both missions maintained the integrity of their decision. Mission A remained convinced that people would not step over the boundaries of salvation if the Islamic teachers were looking over their shoulders. Mission B believed that the walls of hostility separating Muslims from Christians were eroding because its presence and commitment to the community built trust and respect among the Islamic leaders, the community's informal but powerful leaders.

The principles of the kingdom of God, symbolized by *shalom*, prevailed. The people in the community experienced a better quality of life, and benefitted from the justice the mission displayed. The graduates of the school became community leaders, teachers and business people. They could trace their education back to the commitment of mission B, and could commend the mission for its commitment to their community.

Twenty-five years later, Christians in the culture trace the beginning of their conversion process to Mission B's decision to stay after the Islamic teachers came to the school. One indigenous Christian told a story about being thrown into a river because of his faith. He swam back to shore because he knew people at the mission cared for him. Another convert said he remembered that incident, and came to Christ years later because of it. Because of Mission B's decision, the people were educated; the sick were healed; the poor and oppressed were empowered; the Good News was preached; and the kingdom of God was revealed.

NOTES

1. This section is based on Paul G. Hiebert, "Conversion Culture and Conjunctive Categories," *Gospel in Context*, Vol. 1:4 (1978): 24-29.

2. Charles H. Kraft, *Christianity in Culture* (Maryknoll: Orbis Books, 1979), p. 239.

ELEVEN

Transformation:
Moving from signs to symbols

The Lord turned to him and said,
"Go in the strength you have and save Israel out of Midian's hand."

Gideon went in, prepared a young goat . . .
[and] made bread without yeast. . . .
the angel of the Lord touched the meat and the unleavened bread.
Fire flared from the rock, consuming the meat and the bread. . . .

Gideon said to God,
"If you will save Israel by my hand as you have promised—
look, I will place a wool fleece on the threshing floor.
If there is dew only on the fleece and all the ground is dry,
then I will know that you will save Israel by my hand, as you said.". . .
Gideon rose early the next day;
he squeezed the fleece and wrung out the dew . . .

Then Gideon said to God,
"Do not be angry with me.
Let me make just one more request.
Allow me one more test with the fleece.
This time make the fleece dry and the ground covered with dew."
Judges 6:14a, 19-21, 36-39

They dress the wound of my people as though it were not serious.
"Peace, peace," they say, when there is no peace.
Jeremiah 8:11

"Peace I leave with you; my peace I give you.
I do not give to you as the world gives.
Do not let your hearts be troubled and do not be afraid."
John 14:27

"WHAT WISDOM will the fox bring?" wonders Amaguime Dolu, a diviner in the plateau village of Bongo, Mali.¹ Amaguime Dolu is a Dogon diviner who believes fox tracks communicate guidance in some supernatural way. He interprets them to answer the tough questions of life. What does the future hold for the villagers? Will the crops be successful this year? Will prosperity come to this village? The fox tracks reveal the answers to these questions.

In another culture, a mother wonders why her newborn infant is ill. She believes someone with the "evil eye" looked at the infant and cursed him. This illness may be only one manifestation of the curse; the child is likely to have a life of illness and misfortune unless someone can reverse the curse. But can she find the person who sent the curse?

The mother has no choice; she must find the person who placed a curse on her child. When she does so, a diviner whose power is stronger than the power of the person who sent the curse can reverse it.

The mother goes to the village diviner to find out who cursed her child. The diviner fills a bowl full of water. He looks into the bowl and, instead of seeing his reflection, he sees the reflection of the woman who cursed the child. Because the diviner has more power than the woman who sent the curse, he can set the child free.

Looking for signs

In American and European cultures, people also want to know the answers to life's tough questions. They need affirmation for the difficult decisions they are making. They also are looking for signs.

They can find the signs inexpensively by reading any one of the many daily newspapers that carry horoscopes. Horoscopes lead people to believe that the relationships between their birth dates and the positions of the stars determine the course of their lives. If people want more security than a newspaper's price brings, they can hire an astrologer for more personal services.

Palm readers are available in American cultures as they are throughout the world. Palm readers believe that truth is in the lines of a person's palms. The palms of the hands tell such things as how long people will live, if they will gain wealth, and if they will have happy marriages.

The Bible also contains incidents in which people sought or followed divine guidance through what they believed were signs from God. By day, a cloud led the Israelites to the promised land, and a pillar of fire guided them by night. The prophet Isaiah told Ahaz, king of Judah, that God would give a sign about the coming of the Messiah: "The virgin will be with child and will give birth to a son, and will call him Immanuel"

(Isa. 7:14). The experience of Gideon, who put a fleece on the threshing floor, is another sign that is familiar to us.

On concepts, signs and symbols

As shown in Figure 11.1 below, the central thesis of this chapter is that a circular relationship exists between concepts, signs, and symbols. The application of the concept produces signs, and we translate the signs into symbols.

In holistic Christian development, the kingdom of God is the concept; God's redemptive work in creation results in signs that we translate into the symbol, *shalom. Shalom,* in turn, points back to the concept of the kingdom of God.

Before expanding this thesis, I must make some distinctions. We must distinguish symbols from signs, and we must define the different types of signs.

The most important type of sign for our purposes is a theophany. The term literally means an appearance of God. It comes from *theos* and *phania,* the Greek words meaning God showing or appearing. The appearance of God to Moses in the burning bush was a theophany (Exod. 3). The pillars of cloud and fire that guided the Israelite community through the wilderness were also theophanies (Num. 9:15-23). So were

Figure 11.1   The relationship between concepts, signs and symbols

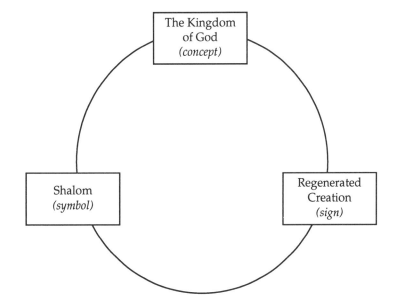

the sightings of the glory of God in the Old Testament (Exod. 33 and Isa. 6). In the New Testament, theophanies are in the forms of doves after the baptism of Jesus, and in "tongues of fire" (Acts 2:3).

The quality that distinguishes theophanies from other types of signs is that the person who experiences them is not directly looking for God to appear. Moses did not seek God in the burning bush, but he was unexpectedly drawn to it. The appearance of the Holy Spirit in the tongues of fire caught the disciples by surprise.

For the purpose of this discussion, two other types of signs are important—general signs and particular signs. People look for both general and particular signs as evidences of God's presence.

A person looks directly for particular signs to reveal the guidance, intervention or presence of God or the supernatural, usually for specific reasons. The Dogon diviner in Mali, the astrologers, palm readers and Gideon are examples of people who seek particular signs.

Particular signs are much more subjective than theophanies, and Scripture—especially the New Testament—does not encourage seeking for them. As Jesus reminds us in the parable of the rich man and Lazarus, particular signs are generally ineffective in helping spiritual growth: "If they do not listen to Moses and the Prophets, they will not be convinced even if someone rises from the dead" (Luke 16:31).

Perhaps Jesus discouraged people from seeking particular signs because particular signs tend to perpetuate the insecurity they are supposed to ease. For example, Gideon received an angel from God telling him that he, Gideon, would lead Israel from the Midianites. The message—a type of theophany—seemed clear, but Gideon proceeded to seek three particular signs to affirm the authenticity of the angel's message.

A pious reading of the Gideon narrative could lead us to believe that Gideon was seeking a sign to confirm each previous sign. But this interpretation is suspect when we read that Gideon was embarrassed to ask for the third sign, and he still remained unconvinced that his calling was genuine. After each sign, the security that Gideon sought so desperately eluded him. Overhearing someone telling a dream about Israel's deliverance from the Midianites finally convinced Gideon that his calling was genuine (Judg. 7:13-15). It was this dream—an unsought sign—not the signs that Gideon sought, that conclusively lead him to accept his calling.

In contrast to particular signs, people do not seek general signs to have God reveal his presence in a particular way or for a specific reason. Instead, they affirm God's presence. Agricultural harvests are examples of general signs. People do not plant crops to bear witness to the particular presence of God, but the harvests point to a Creator who works redemptively in an environment that is conducive to agricultural harvests.

When the Corinthians questioned Paul's credibility, he used general signs to support his apostleship. He reminded the Corinthians that signs, wonders and miracles were done among them (2 Cor. 12:12). Apparently, the specific reasons for these signs were not to convince the Corinthians of God's call on Paul. However, Paul expected the signs, wonders and miracles to bear witness—in a general way—to the authenticity of his calling to be an apostle.

Definition of symbols

Symbols differ from signs. They are not evidences of the concepts they represent. Instead, we create symbols from signs to bear witness to the concepts from which the signs resulted. If we think of signs as evidences of events that occurred in a particular space and time, symbols reflect that event over space and time.

Words are our most common symbols. They make the concepts that are apparent in signs intelligible, accessible and communicable. The word *time* is a good example. It represents a concept we can understand, and we can find signs that show that time exists. Yet communicating the concept—or even the sign—is cumbersome until we bring the concept and the signs together in a symbol, the word *time*.

Symbols also enable us to communicate abstract concepts that are relative to cultures effectively. People frequently use animals to symbolize qualities that are difficult to communicate. American English uses the fox to communicate the concepts of cunningness and slyness, the owl to symbolize wisdom, and the rabbit to symbolize fertility. In other cultures, the fox is a symbol of treachery,[2] and the owl is a symbol of evil or witchcraft. In each situation, the symbol provides a visual image for a more abstract concept.

Holidays also become symbols that result from signs. Christmas and Easter are two Christian holidays that symbolize the birth and resurrection of Christ. Individual countries and cultures also have holidays to symbolize noteworthy religious, political, social and cultural signs.

Symbols are particularly helpful in making the presence of God discernible, intelligible or accessible. In contrast to signs, we do not use symbols as evidences of God's presence. Through symbols, however, people receive the affirmation that God is present. At the baptism of Jesus, a dove communicated the descent of the Holy Spirit. The dove was a sign that has since become a symbol of the Holy Spirit.

Other signs have also become symbols. The fire on the altar in the temple was a symbol of God's presence (Lev. 6:12-13). It reminded people of the times when God had actually appeared in fire and, because it burned constantly, it pointed toward God's constant presence. We continue to use candles in worship to symbolize the presence of God.

The meanings of symbols change between cultures and over time

The meanings of signs and symbols are not static, but change over time and between cultures. As shown above, the fox as a symbol has different meanings in different cultures; the holiday, Pentecost, does as well. In the Christian calendar, Pentecost, which means 50, is the birthday of the church. It happened fifty days after Passover, and symbolizes the day when the Holy Spirit inaugurated the new religious movement by descending upon believers.

In the Hebrew calendar, Pentecost is the Feast of Weeks, or the Day of First Fruits. It was an agricultural holiday that marked the conclusion of Passover, and commemorated the end of the harvest season. We can find signs and symbols, such as the end of Passover and the offerings of first fruits, that symbolize the transition of the holiday from the Hebrew to the Christian calendar. Even so, the holiday in the two cultures remains distinct.

The transformation of fish from signs of deity in various ancient Middle Eastern religions to symbols of Christianity is also worth examining to understand how people transform symbols cross-culturally. In ancient cultures, fish were either general or particular signs, theophanies or intrinsically divine beings. They eventually became enduring symbols of Christianity. Christians today, like their first and second century spiritual ancestors, display fish as symbols of their commitment to believing and communicating "Jesus Christ, Son of God, Savior." (The Greek word for fish, ICTHUS, forms an acrostic from the Greek words meaning Jesus Christ, Son of God, Savior.)

Christians who are unfamiliar with ancient Middle Eastern religious signs probably believe that the early Christians developed the symbol of the fish around the acrostic, ICTHUS. Yet the opposite is probably true. The fish as a sacred sign was so common "that one gets the impression that everyone in the first century was a devotee of the sacred fish, under one form or another."[3] Undoubtedly, a first or second century Christian scribe noticed ICTHUS formed an acrostic for the central theological statement of his faith. In appropriating and displaying the symbol, early Christians—unlike their contemporaries from other religions—did not believe the fish were "fit to be venerated."[4] Instead, they were showing how signs in one culture can become symbols in another.

Besides changing from one culture to another, symbols within the culture also change over time. The American celebration of Thanksgiving is a good example. It began as a feast to honor God for his blessing of an abundant harvest. As the years passed, Americans continued to celebrate the holiday in thanksgiving to God, but this meaning has become secondary. The churches in the United States do not generally hold worship services on Thanksgiving, and people spend the day eating and watching football games. If people who do not live in the American culture could observe Thanksgiving, they probably would not associate it with a religious celebration.

Pentecost is another example of a holiday that had its meaning changed over time. While it changed meanings from the Hebrew to the Christian calendar, it also changed its meaning within the Hebrew calendar. As mentioned above, it began as an agricultural festival, a meaning the Hebrews kept until about 200 A.D. After that date, it became a holiday to commemorate the giving of the Torah. The Hebrews transformed the Feast of Weeks from a celebration of the end of the seven-week growing season to celebrating the "courting days of the bridegroom Israel with the bride Torah."[5]

Transforming signs, symbols and world views

While people commonly use signs to seek God's will, or to discern supernatural intervention in nature, they pose a challenge for practitioners of holistic Christian development. We must identify the signs that reflect the nature of our work, and we must transform them into one or more symbols. We should develop symbols that communicate the entire scope of our work in relation to God's redemptive work in creation.

This process of transforming signs into symbols is parallel to the transformation of primal or Western world views into a holistic, biblical world view. Signs and symbols are apparent in both world views, but they do not necessarily reflect the signs and symbols of holistic Christian development.

In cultures with primal world views, for example, signs might include trees, animals, and a variety of natural formations. The idea that the spiritual realm dictates the actions of the physical realm precludes the possibility that nature is random. Things don't just happen—they happen for a specific reason. Therefore, we can interpret the lines of a person's palms, an animal sighting, and animal tracks as meaningful signs. For example, the sighting of an animal over a person's grave says something about the spiritual power of the person.

Signs in primal cultures are likely to have a negative effect on the development process. People who seek such signs are not likely to be innovative or to think developmentally. They are more likely to resist developmental innovations because of their fear of the spiritual realm.

The fear works itself out in two vital expressions. As mentioned in previous chapters, people fear a change of traditions because they do not wish to offend the spiritual realm. People are particularly afraid of offending their ancestors if they change their traditional ways.

A second expression of fear is the social and spiritual alienation that can result from success. People in primal communities can possibly attribute a person's success to sorcery. Since the people define themselves in relation to their community, they understand this practice as one person jeopardizing the welfare of the entire community for individual gain. The risk of being accused of sorcery is not worth the benefits of success. A recent report from the Human Social Research Council supports this belief. It reads:

> In recent years, the homeland [Venda, South Africa] has seen a rise in secret ritual killings of individuals, such as businessmen seeking to improve their personal fortunes. . . . If a businessman or farmer prospers, he risks being accused of witchcraft. In one case, an agriculture official retired and returned to his old village. Because he used modern farming techniques, his crops flourished. Neighbors accused him of using zombies, the living dead, to tend his fields at night. He was burned to death.[6]

Such incidents will probably lead people away from God's call to work actively toward implementing projects that are developmental or innovative. People are more comfortable as passengers in the back of a truck; they are unwilling to chart the course of their lives, but passively accept the status quo as the will of the spiritual realm. They believe they are helpless to affect the will of the spiritual realm.

Development and spirituality

In cultures where people have modern, theistic world views, the problems of development are opposite from those in primal cultures. People from modern, theistic cultures believe development negatively affects the spirituality of a people or a culture. In this world view, the spiritual realm does not dictate the physical realm. Instead, people who hold this world view believe the physical realm is autonomous from any spiritual influence. This creates the problem of understanding the influence of the spiritual realm in holistic Christian development.

Development perpetuates this problem. People do not directly attribute to God their ability to manipulate physical elements so they can increase agricultural harvests or treat illnesses. Instead, they see development as the result of social or scientific innovations.

More often than not, these innovations have a secularizing effect on cultures. People do not believe the innovations bear witness to the inspiration of God. Instead, the innovations create the problem of fitting God into the scientific presuppositions that produce the innovations. The people ask: How is God relevant to the modern world? What is God's place in science? Is healing from God or from medical technology?

In the Western world view, questions concerning God and development, or the scientific or technological innovations that people use in development, are generally answered in an either-or fashion. Since Westerners do not believe in the interaction of the physical and spiritual realms, God's role in development is not obvious. The challenge, therefore, is to transform the world views of the people so that they see God effecting changes in the physical environment.

Signs in the modern, theistic world view perpetuate the belief in the separation of the physical and spiritual realms. General signs—those that show the natural changes in the environment—are not directly attributed to God. People can explain them by the interaction of physical elements in the universe. Plants grow, not because God intervenes, but because soils, fertilizer and water interact to enable seeds to germinate.

If people interpret signs in the physical realm as interventions from God or the supernatural realm, these signs indicate the exceptional times when the spiritual realm crosses the boundaries of the physical-spiritual dichotomy. People consider such signs miraculous or mysterious, but this is a tentative conclusion: they are supernatural until natural explanations can be found.

In this world view, people perceive that God has different roles in development. Some people will say that God does not influence changes in the physical world. Instead, God influences the interpretations that enable us to understand physical changes.

This view does not see God as the source of the changes, but as the factor that enables us to place a value on the changes. If we can place a value on the changes, then God must influence our values simply because our fallen nature prevents us from making valid value judgements. If we carry this view to its logical extent, we believe God influences development ethics, and inspires values we communicate through development, but his activity is not in the actual work.

People who are not satisfied to see God's work in the interpretation of an event are vulnerable to seeing that God's work fills the gaps of life. This understanding of God's work is known as "God of the gaps." It states that God will fill the gaps in the physical realm that emerge when we reach the limits of human ability, managerial competence, or physical resources. If God chooses not to intervene and bridge the gaps, then development has no intrinsic Christian witness.

Shalom as a symbol of holistic Christian development

Holistic Christian development transforms the presuppositions of both the Western and primal world views by incorporating the signs of development into the symbol of *shalom*. Holistic Christian development does not perceive God's role as that of filling gaps. Instead, it proposes that *shalom* symbolizes the presence of a Creator who works to restore the entire creation to fulfill the purposes for which he created it. To this extent, people see the presence of God in ordinary situations. He brings meaning to meaninglessness.

In representing the redemption of the entire creation, *shalom* makes development intrinsically evangelistic. Besides transforming general signs to bear witness to God's presence in regenerating creation, holism gives people the assurance they seek in particular signs. They do not have to cope with the insecurity or subjectivity of finding God's will through particular signs within themselves or their environments. Instead, they can measure choices against the ability of these choices to produce *shalom*.

Using *shalom* as a symbol of Christian ministry, though, raises the issue of expanding its common meaning to incorporate all the facets of life in the kingdom of God. Currently, the term suffers from narrow perceptions and definitions. We proclaim Jesus as the "Prince of Peace," but we are more prone to thinking of this peace as a feeling of inner, personal or individual contentment, instead of believing it communicates a sense of harmony in creation. We do not think peace symbolizes the way of life in God's kingdom, or the sense of wholeness in creation that results from the reconciliation of creation to the Creator.

Our narrow definition of *shalom* should make us redefine it so we can communicate the conviction that holism, through *shalom*, makes development holy. A model of holistic Christian development based on *shalom* does not support the idea that development is "based on the implicit belief that human society is inevitably progressing toward the attainment of a temporal materialistic kingdom."[7] Instead, a development model based on *shalom* suggests that material growth is necessary to the point where it enables people to experience the abundant life we have in Christ. People who suffer from material deprivation do not have peace in a holistic sense.

Shalom, in its purest form, is a transcultural and timeless concept. Yet like other symbols, its meaning is subject to change over time and between cultures. Like Pentecost—a symbol whose meaning has changed over time—and the fish—a symbol whose meaning has changed between cultures—the meaning of *shalom* is expanded and transformed as people understand and experience God's redemptive work in a culture. *Shalom*

Figure 11.2   Hebraic-Holistic world view[8]

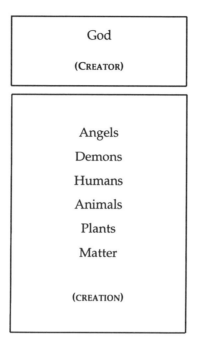

will have different expressions as cultures move toward fuller realizations of justice, righteousness, salvation and wholeness.

If we see Christian mission responding to a holistic view of creation (see Figure 11.2 above), we can more easily envision *shalom* as a symbol that is born out of God's redemptive work in creation. This world view does not create the dichotomy that results from a Western world view, or integrate God into nature as the primal world view does. Instead, it recognizes that God's uncreated nature separates him from creation, and enables us to focus on the redemptive work of God in creation.

In the biblical holistic world view, we do not classify the disciplines we use in Christian development according to their spiritual or physical natures. Instead, we value these disciplines for the contributions they make toward the redemption of creation. We transform Figure 11.3 to Figure 11.4 (see page 174), rendering the dichotomies of the modern theistic world view meaningless. Such distinctions as spiritual-physical, supernatural-natural, sacred-secular, values-facts, or private-public fail to define the nature of the disciplines, or the spheres in which we use them.

For example, we cannot separate the values of the social and physical sciences from their facts. The very nature of the disciplines requires

Figure 11.3   The spiritual-physical dichotomy

Spiritual
(supernatural, sacred, values, private)

Theology
Religion
Ethics
Christian Education

(*Evangelism*)

Physical
(natural, secular, facts, public)

Physical Sciences
Social Sciences
Economics
Management
Secular Education

(*Development*)

Figure 11.4   Holistic view of the disciplines used in Christian development

Holism

Theology
Religion
Ethics
Physical Sciences
Social Sciences

some level of interpretation; interpretation involves values. In this regard, the ethical perspectives that Christianity brings to the principles of the disciplines are not mere appendages. Instead, Christian ethics transforms the values we currently use in the disciplines to focus the disciplines on *shalom*.

In medicine, the emphasis of treatment is not on natural cures in the absence of supernatural cures. Instead, a holistic Christian perspective sees God as the source of all healing. This does not mean we can discount the idea that God can intervene in nature to hasten healing. Instead, we can attribute all healing to God because God created systems within creation that facilitate healing.

Christian holism calls us to consider the fuller dimension of God's plan for salvation. When the ancient Hebrews spoke of *shalom* they communicated the idea that life in creation under the sovereignty of God was all right. They envisioned "a state of wholeness possessed by persons or groups which [included] health, prosperity, security, or the completeness of the covenant."[9] People did not have to reconcile their spiritual comfort in the midst of physical despair. Such a reconciliation would have been foreign to people who did not distinctly separate the physical and spiritual dimensions of their beings.

Yet *shalom*'s qualities do not characterize the world we face. Twenty percent of the world's population are homeless, 40 percent are hungry, and the few wealthy people in the world are rendering the poor economically powerless. If we do not grasp the full implications of *shalom*, then we—the blessed peacemakers who serve the Prince of Peace—will communicate a hollow message. We will be like the prophets Jeremiah confronted, who proclaimed, "Peace, peace" when there was no peace (Jer. 8:11). At that time, the kingdom of Judah was on the verge of collapse.

The peace of Christ is unlike the peace of this world. It is an everlasting peace that communicates the hope creation has in the regenerative work of Christ. It is a peace that we proclaim in everything we do and all that we are. It calls us:

> *. . . to preach good news to the poor.*
> *. . . proclaim freedom for the prisoners*
> *and recovery of sight for the blind,*
> *to release the oppressed,*
> *to proclaim the year of the Lord's favor.*
> *Luke 4:18-19*

NOTES

1. David Roberts, "Mali's Dogon People: Below the Cliff of Tombs," *National Geographic*, Vol. 178:4, pp. 104-105.

2. Charles H. Kraft, *Christianity in Culture: A Study in Dynamic Biblical Theologizing in Cross-Cultural Perspective* (Maryknoll: Orbis Books, 1979), p. 132.

3. Cyril C. Richardson, "The Foundations of Christian Symbolism," *Religious Symbolism* (New York: Harper and Row, 1955), p. 6.

4. Ibid., p. 5.

5. J.C. Rylaarsdam, "Weeks, Feast of," *Interpreter's Dictionary of the Bible*, Vol. 4, George Buttrick, ed. (New York: Abingdon Press, 1964), p. 828.

6. Greg Myer, "Witchcraft Roils South African Politics," *Los Angeles Times* (April 12, 1992), p. A12.

7. Tom Sine, "Development: Its Secular Past and Its Uncertain Future," *The Church in Response to Human Need* (Monrovia: MARC, 1983), p. 22.

8. Paul G. Hiebert, *Phenomenology and Institutions of Folk Religions* (Pasadena: Fuller Theological Seminary, 1990), p. 22.

9. E.M. Good, "Peace in the Old Testament," *Interpreter's Dictionary of the Bible*, Vol. 3, George Buttrick, ed. (New York: Abingdon Press, 1964), pp. 705-706.

Selected Bibliography

Allen, Diogenes. *Christian Belief in a Postmodern World: The Full Wealth of Conviction*. Louisville: Westminster/John Knox Press, 1989.

_____. *Philosophy for Understanding Theology*. Atlanta: John Knox Press, 1985.

Barbour, Ian G. *Science and Secularity: The Ethics of Technology*. New York: Harper and Row, 1970.

Barrett, David B. *Schism and Renewal in Africa: An Analysis of Six Thousand Contemporary Religious Movements*. New York: Oxford University Press, 1968.

Berger, Peter L. *A Rumor of Angels: Modern Society and the Rediscovery of the Supernatural*. Garden City: Doubleday & Company, 1969.

_____. *The Sacred Canopy: Elements of a Sociological Theory of Religion*. Garden City: Doubleday & Company, 1967.

Bonk, Jon. "'All Things to All Persons'—The Missionary as a Racist-Imperialist, 1860-1918". *Missiology: An International Review*, Vol. 8:3, 1980.

Bosch, David J. *Transforming Mission: Paradigm Shifts in Theology of Mission*. Maryknoll: Orbis Books, 1991.

Brown, Robert McAfee. *Making Peace in the Global Village*. Philadelphia: The Westminster Press, 1981.

Buju, Benezet. *African Theology in its Social Context*. Maryknoll: Orbis Books, 1992.

Burnett, David. *Clash of Worlds*. Eastbourne: MARC/Monarch Publications, Ltd., 1990.

_____. *Unearthly Powers: A Christian Perspective on Primal and Folk Religions*. Eastbourne, UK: MARC/Monarch Publications, Ltd., 1988.

Butterfield, Herbert. *The Origins of Modern Science: 1300-1800*. New York: MacMillan, 1962.

Buttrick, George, editor. *The Interpreter's Dictionary of the Bible*, Vol. 1-4. New York: Abingdon Press, 1964.

Chambers, Robert. *Rural Development: Putting the Last First*. Essex: Longman Group, Ltd., 1983.

Cross, Nigel and Riannon Barker. *At the Desert's Edge: Oral Histories from the Sahel*. London: Panos Publications, 1992.

Curle, Adam. *Education for Liberation*. London: Tavistock Publications, 1973.

Daniels, Nomsa. "Guardians of Eden." *African Report*, Sept.-Oct. 1991.

Davis, John Jefferson. *Your Wealth in God's World: Does the Bible Support the Free Market?* Phillipsburg: Presbyterian and Reformed Publishing Co., 1984.

Denffer, Dietrich Von. "Baraka as a Basic Concept of Muslim Popular Belief." *Islamic Studies*, 15:167-186, 1976.

de Rosny, Eric. *Healers in the Night*. Maryknoll: Orbis Books, 1985.

Duchrow, Ulrich & Gerhard Liedke. *Shalom: Biblical Perspectives on Creation, Justice & Peace*. Geneva: WCC Publications, 1987.

Dyrness, William A. *Learning about Theology from the Third World*. Grand Rapids: Zondervan, 1990.

_____. *Let the Earth Rejoice: A Biblical Theology of Holistic Mission*. Westchester: Crossway Books, 1983.

Eboussi, Boulaga F. *Christianity without Fetishes: A Critique and Recapture of Christianity*. Maryknoll: Orbis, 1984.

Eliade, Mircea. *The Sacred and the Profane: The Nature of Religion*. Translated by Williard Trask. New York: Harcourt Brace, 1959.

Elliston, Edgar J., editor. *Christian Relief and Development: Developing Workers for Christian Ministry*. Dallas: Word, Inc., 1989.

Evans, Robert A., and Heidi Hadsell de Nascimento. "Ecologists and the Rain Forest." *The Christian Century*, Vol. 108:32, Nov. 6, 1991.

Ewert, D. Merrill, editor. *A New Agenda for Medical Missions*. Brunswick: MAP International, 1990.

Ewert, Norm. "The Role of Business Enterprise in Christian Mission." *Transformation*, Vol. 9:1, 1992.

Fountain, Daniel E. *Health, the Bible and the Church*. Wheaton: The Billy Graham Center, 1989.

Freire, Paulo. *Pedagogy of the Oppressed*. New York: Continuum Publishing Co., 1986.

Gehman, Richard. "African Religion Lives." *Evangelical Missions Quarterly*, Vol. 27:4, 1991.

Gilliland, Dean S., editor. *The Word Among Us: Contextualizing Theology for Mission Today*. Dallas: Word Publishing, 1989.

Goulet, Denis S. *The Uncertain Promise: Values Conflict in Technology Transfer*. New York: New Horizons Press, 1989.

Granberg-Michaelson, Wesley, editor. *Tending the Garden: Essays on the Gospel and the Earth*. Grand Rapids: Wm. B. Eerdmans Publishing Co., 1987.

Grollig, Francis X., S.J., and Francis B. Haley, editors. *Medical Anthropology*. The Hague: Mouton Publishers, 1976.

Haring, Bernard. *The Healing Power of Peace and Non-Violence*. New York: Paulist Press, 1986.

Harris, Marvin. *Cows, Pigs, Wars and Witches: The Riddles of Culture*. New York: Vintage Books, 1974.

Hay, Donald A. *Economics Today: A Christian Critique*. Leicester: Apollos Press, 1989.

Henry, Carl F.H. and Robert Lincoln Hancock, editors. *The Ministry of Development in Evangelical Perspective*. Pasadena: Wm. Carey Library, 1979.

Hess, Robert. "Wholeness and Health in Contemporary Nigeria." *Missiology: An International Review*, Vol. 11:2, April 1983.

Hiebert, Paul G. and Frances F., editors. *Case Studies in Missions*. Grand Rapids: Baker Book House, 1987.

Hiebert, Paul G. "Spiritual Warfare: An Anabaptist Perspective." *Mission Focus*, Vol. 20:3, 1992.

_____. "From Neo-Colonialism to Globalism." *Missiology: An International Review*, Vol. 19:3, 1991.

_____. *Phenomenology and Institutions of Folk Religions*. Pasadena: Fuller Theological Seminary, 1990.

_____. "Healing and the Kingdom," *Wonders and the Word*. Manitoba: Kindred Press, 1989.

_____. "Power Encounter and Folk Islam," *Muslims and Christians on the Emmaus Road*. Edited by J. Dudley Woodberry. Monrovia: MARC, 1989.

_____. "Critical Contextualization." *International Bulletin of Missions Research*, Vol. 11:3, 1987.

_____. "Critical Contextualization." *Missiology: An International Review*, Vol. 12:3, 1984.

_____. "The Category 'Christian' in the Mission Task." *International Review of Missions*, Vol. 72:287, 1983.

_____. "The Bicultural Bridge." *Mission Focus*, Vol. 10:1, 1982.

_____. "The Flaw of the Excluded Middle." *Missiology: An International Review*, Vol. 10:1, 1982.

_____. "Conversion, Culture and Cognitive Categories." *Gospel in Context*, Vol. 1:4, 1978.

_____. "Traffic Patterns in Seattle and Hyderabad: Immediate and Mediate Transactions." *Journal of Anthropological Research*, University of New Mexico, Vol. 32:4, 1976.

Heilbroner, Robert L. *The Worldly Philosophers*. New York: Simon and Schuster, 1986.

Hovey, Kevin G. *Before All Else Fails . . . Read the Directions*. Brisbane: Harvest Publications, 1986.

Isbister, John. *Promises Not Kept: The Betrayal of Social Change in the Third World*. West Hartford: Kumarian Press, 1992.

Joedhiswara, Mikha. "Holistic Evangelism: On Suffering in the Face of Overwhelming Poverty and Multifaced Religiosity." *Mission Focus*, Vol. 20:2, 1992.

Johnson, F. Ernest, editor. *Religious Symbolism*. New York: Harper and Row, 1955.

Joranson, Philip N. and Ken Butigen. *The Cry of the Environment: Rebuilding the Christian Creation Tradition*. Santa Fe: Bear Publications, 1984.

Kelsey, Morton T. *Psychology, Medicine and Christian Healing*. New York: Harper and Row, 1988.

_____. *Myth, History and Faith: The Remythologization of Christianity*. New York: Paulist Press, 1974.

Kenyon, John A. "Toward the light of literacy." *Together*, Vol. 29:1-2, 1991.

_____. "How shall we care for the earth." *Together*, Vol. 21:1-2, 1989.

Klem, Herbert V. *Oral Communication of the Scripture*. Pasadena: William Carey Library, 1982.

Korten, David C. *Getting to the 21st Century: Voluntary Action and the Global Agenda*. W. Hartford: Kumarian Press, Inc., 1990.

Kraft, Charles H. *Christianity with Power: Your Worldview and Your Experience of the Supernatural*. Ann Arbor: Servant Books, 1989.

_____. *Christianity in Culture: A Study in Dynamic Biblical Theologizing in Cross-*

Cultural Perspective. Maryknoll: Orbis Books, 1979.

Lane, Belden C. "The Power of Myth: Lessons from Joseph Campbell." *The Christian Century*, Vol. 106, July 5-12, 1989.

Libreros, Augusto. "Expressing Christian Solidarity." *Together*, Vol. 30, 1991.

Leibrecht, Water, editor. *Religion and Culture: Essays in Honor of Paul Tillich.* New York: Harper and Brothers, 1959.

Linthicum, Robert C. *Empowering the Poor: Community organizing among the city's "rag, tag and bobtail."* Monrovia: MARC, 1991.

Luscombe, Kenneth L. "Discipleship as a Paradigm for Health, Healing and Wholeness." *Health, Healing and Transformation.* E. Anthony Allen, et al. Monrovia: MARC/WVI, 1991.

Mabudiga, Nzunga. *Some Implications of Indigenous Healing for the Christian Church in Zaire.* D. Min. thesis, Eastern Baptist Theological Seminary, 1980.

Malinowski, Bronislaw. *Magic, Science and Religion and other Essays.* New York: Anchor Books, 1954.

Mauser, Ulrich. *The Gospel of Peace: A Scriptural Message for Today's World.* Louisville: Westminster/John Knox Press, 1992.

McDonagh, Sean. *To Care for the Earth.* London: Geoffrey Chapman, 1986.

Meeks, M. Douglas. *God the Economist: The Doctrine of God and Political Economy.* Minneapolis: Augsburg Press, 1989.

Metzler, James E. *From Saigon to Shalom.* Scottdale: Herald Press, 1985.

Meyer, Art & Jocele. *Earthkeepers: Environmental Perspectives on Hunger, Poverty & Injustice.* Scottdale: Herald Press, 1991.

Mikulencak, Ruby. "Science and Magic Collide in African Medicine." *Evangelical Missions Quarterly*, Vol. 23:4, 1987.

Mott, Stephen Charles. *Biblical Ethics and Social Change.* New York: Oxford University Press, 1982.

Musk, Bill A. *The Unseen Face of Islam: Sharing the Gospel with Ordinary Muslims.* Eastbourne: MARC/Monarch Publications, Ltd., 1989.

Myers, Bryant L. "The Sacrament of Well Drilling." *MARC Newsletter*, No. 90-3, 1990.

Myers, David G. *The Human Puzzle: Psychological Research and Christian Belief.* New York: Harper and Row, 1978.

Newbigin, Lesslie. *The Gospel in a Pluralist Society.* Grand Rapids: Wm. B. Eerdmans, 1989.

_____. "Response to David M. Stowe." *International Bulletin of Missionary Research*, Vol. 12:4, Oct. 1988.

_____. "Can the West be Converted?" *International Bulletin of Missionary Research*, Vol. 11:1, 1987.

_____. *Honest Religion for Secular Man*. Philadelphia: Westminster Press, 1966.

Ramseyer, Robert L., editor. *Mission and the Peace Witness*. Scottdale: Herald Press, 1979.

Remenyi, Joe V. *Where Credit Is Due: Income-Generating Programmes for the Poor in Developing Countries*. London: Intermediate Technology Publications, 1991.

Riddle, Norman G., *Unreached People Survey* (Zaire). Unpublished paper.

Sanneh, Lamin. "Christian Missions and the Western Guilt Complex." *The Christian Century*, April 8, 1987.

Schumacher, E.F. *Good Work*. New York: Harper and Row, 1979.

_____. *Small is Beautiful: Economics as if People Mattered*. New York: Harper and Row, 1973.

Shorter, Aylward. *Jesus and the Witchdoctor: Approaches to Healing and Wholeness*. Maryknoll: Orbis Press, 1985.

_____. *African Culture and the Christian Church*. Maryknoll: Orbis Press, 1973.

Sider, Ronald J. *Rich Christians in an Age of Hunger*. Dallas: Word Publishing, 1990.

_____. *Evangelicals and Development: Toward a Theology of Social Change*. Philadelphia: Westminster Press, 1981.

Sine, Tom, editor. *The Church in Response to Human Need*. Monrovia: MARC, 1983.

Smart, Ninian. *Worldviews: Cross-cultural Exploration of Human Beliefs*. New York: Scribners, 1983.

Steyne, Philip M. *Gods of Power: A Study of the Beliefs and Practices of Animists*, Houston: Touch Publications, 1990.

Stott, John R.W. *Christian Missions in the Modern World*. Downers Grove: Inter-Varsity Press, 1975.

Stowe, David M. "Modernization and Resistance: Theological Implications for Mission." *International Bulletin of Missionary Research*, Vol. 12:4, 1988.

Stromberg, J.A., n.d. *The Christian Concept of Healing* (unpublished paper).

Tam, Michael L. "Primary Health Care and Indigenous Medicine." *Cultural Survival Quarterly*, 12:1, 1988.

Teeter, David. "Dynamic Equivalent Conversion for Tentative Muslim Believers." *Missiology: An International Review*, 18:3, 1990.

Todaro, Michael P. *Economic Development in the Third World*, 4th Ed. White Plains: Longman Press, 1989.

Wakatama, Pius. *Independence for the Third World Church: An African's Perspective on Missionary Work*. Downer's Grove: InterVarsity Press, 1976.

Warner, Paula. "African Healer vs Missionary Physician." *Evangelical Missions Quarterly*, Vol. 26:4, 1990.

West, Charles C. "Mission to the West: A Dialogue with Stowe and Newbigin." *International Bulletin of Missionary Research*, Vol. 12:4, 1988.

Wink, Walter. *Unmasking the Powers: The Invisible Forces That Determine Human Existence*. Philadelphia: Fortress Press, 1986.

_____. *Engaging the Powers*. Minneapolis: Augsburg Fortress Press, 1992.

Wolters, Albert M. *Creation Regained: Biblical Basis for a Reformational Worldview*. Grand Rapids: Wm. B. Eerdmans, 1985.

Wolterstorff, Nicholas. *Until Justice & Peace Embrace*. Grand Rapids: Wm. B. Eerdmans, 1983.

Woodward, Kenneth L., et al. "Talking to God." *Newsweek*, January 6, 1992.

Yoder, John Howard. *The Politics of Jesus*. Grand Rapids: Wm. B. Eerdmans, 1972.

Yoder, P. Stanley, editor. *African Health and Healing Systems: Proceedings of a Symposium*. Los Angeles: Crossroads Press, 1982.

Yohannan, K.P. *Why the World Waits: Exposing the Reality of Modern Missions*. Lake Mary: Creation House, 1991.

Yost, Jim. "Development work can hinder church growth." *Evangelical Missions Quarterly*, 1984

Young, David, et al. "The Persistence of Traditional Medicine in the Modern World." *Cultural Survival Quarterly*, Vol. 12:1, 1988.

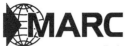

MARC

Bringing you key resources on the world mission of the church

MARC books and other publications support the work of MARC (Mission Advanced Research and Communications Center), which is to inspire fresh vision and empower the Christian mission among those who extend the whole gospel to the whole world.

Recent MARC titles include:

▶ *Women as Leaders* by Katherine Haubert. Scrutinizes Scripture to help the reader come to his or her own conclusions about the contemporary reality of women leaders in the church and ministry. Formatted to facilitate easy group or individual study.   E-013 $8.95

▶ *Mission Handbook 1993-95*. The 1993-95 edition continues as the most comprehensive listing available of Christian mission agencies based in North America, with detailed up-to-date descriptions and statistics, analyses and essays. Also available in a powerful IBM-compatible computer software version.

Mission Handbook plus *Mission Handbook on Disk*	A-016b	$119.95
Mission Handbook on Disk (software only)	A-016d	$ 99.95
Mission Handbook 1993-95 (book only)	A-016	$ 39.95

▶ *The Changing Shape of World Mission* by Bryant L. Myers. Presents in color graphics the challenge before missions globally, including the unfinished task of world evangelization.   A-017 $5.95

▶ *I Sing of Hope* by Valdir R. Steuernagel. A Latin American examines Psalm 146 in tandem with Mary's *Magnificat* and invites the reader to transform the passages into a program of action.   R-006 $4.95

Order Toll Free in USA: **1-800-777-7752**
Visa and MasterCard accepted

MARC

A division of World Vision International
121 E. Huntington Drive
Monrovia, CA 91016-3400

Ask for the MARC Newsletter and complete publications list